THE NATURAL WAY

Diabetes

Catherine Steven

Series medical consultants
Dr Peter Albright MD (USA)
& Dr David Peters MD (UK)

Approved by the
AMERICAN HOLISTIC MEDICAL ASSOCIATION
& BRITISH HOLISTIC MEDICAL ASSOCIATION

E L E M E N T
Shaftesbury, Dorset ● Boston, Massachusetts
Melbourne, Australia

© Element Books Limited 1995
Text © Catherine Steven 1995

First Published in the UK in 1995 by
Element Books Limited
Shaftesbury, Dorset SP7 8BP

Published in the USA in 1995 by
Element Books, Inc.
160 North Washington Street, Boston, MA 02114

Published in Australia in 1995 by
Element Books
and distributed by
Penguin Australia Limited
487 Maroondah Highway, Ringwood, Victoria 3134

Reissued 1998
Reprinted 1999

Cover design by Slatter-Anderson
Designed and typeset by Linda Reed and Joss Nizan
Printed and bound in Great Britain

British Library Cataloguing in Publication
data available

Library of Congress Cataloguing in Publication Data
Steven, Catherine, 1956-
The natural way with diabetes/Catherine Steven.
    p.   cm. -- (The Natural way series)
Includes bibliographical references and index.
ISBN 1–85230–705-6 (pbk.)
1. Diabetes-Alternative treatment. 2. Holistic medicine.
I. title. II. Series.
RC660.S734 1995
616.4′62–dc20   95–30817
CIP

ISBN 1 85230 705 6

Contents

Illustrations

For Babis, George and Nikki, naturally

Acknowledgements

My thanks to everyone who helped provide information about diabetes for this book. In particular to Andrew Ozanne, who made a lot possible at a crucial stage, George Oswald and Anne Kinch for their time and patience, Katy Griggs, a mine of information, Prof Edwin Gale, Prof David Barker, Nick London, Christopher Bennetto, Dr John Stanley, Dr Peter Ellis for his enthusiasm and guidance, and last but not least the parents of diabetics, and the adult diabetics who gave me their own personal insight into this most complex and challenging disease.

Introduction

Over 100 million people around the world have diabetes – nearly a third of the total in Europe alone – and according to the International Diabetes Federation we are in the grip of a global epidemic. The number of diagnosed cases has tripled in the past eight years and more are recognized with each and every passing year.

We are all at risk, for diabetes can strike without warning in any family, at any time.

Diabetes is a disease of the Western world, rare in rural Africa, most common in Northern Europe and America and there are strong associations with an affluent lifestyle. Northern European countries have the highest rates of the disease anywhere in the world.

Indeed, in Europe the incidence has doubled in the past 20 years and it is now recognized as one of the fastest growing childhood diseases. For children, diabetes means a lifetime on medication, and a higher than average risk of kidney or heart disease later in life.

Many people have diabetes and don't know it until the symptoms of the disease become so acute they need urgent medical attention. In America diabetes affects nearly one in 20, and is the third biggest killer above lung and breast cancer. One in five Americans can now expect to develop diabetes, if they live into their seventies.

Although the statistics look grim, and they are, we can take action to combat this killer disease of the so-called developed world.

Living with diabetes largely means taking matters into your own hands, dealing with it on a day-to-day basis. This book does not hold the answers to curing diabetes – for there is no cure. But with careful management, and the right help and guidance it is possible to use safe and gentle methods to *manage* diabetes in a natural, healthy, and rejuvenating way.

With the right diet, and innovative new ideas from food scientists – explored in this book – many diabetics should be able to manage their diabetes without any form of medication.

As a diabetic you may face some resistance to 'natural therapies' from your conventional family practitioner. But by introducing safe therapies such as stress management, or relaxation and exercise therapies such as yoga, which lower blood glucose levels, it *is* possible to improve your overall sense of wellbeing. Positive health for diabetics means keeping the disease on an even keel without unnatural highs and lows.

The most natural way with this extraordinarily complex disease, however, has to be prevention. In most cases there is a period of decline towards diabetes several years before the symptoms become so acute that treatment is essential for survival.

There is a growing awareness of how we all might arm ourselves against diabetes through improved diet, exercise and a healthier lifestyle.

The key to good health lies in the hands of diabetics themselves and this book is dedicated to all who are diabetics, or who are on the brink of the disease (but have not yet toppled over the edge), and are prepared to take life in both hands and do something to help themselves . . . positively, but above all naturally.

CHAPTER 1

What is diabetes?

How it develops and who is affected

Diabetes – or *diabetes mellitus* to give it its proper medical name – is one of the oldest and most complex diseases known to humankind. Mentioned as early as 1500 BC in Egyptian papyrus scrolls (a high fibre diet of wheat grains and ochre was recommended), the condition was first described as diabetes by the Ancient Greek physician Aretaeus of Cappadocia in 100 AD. He described the life of its victims as 'short and painful'.

The word *diabetes* originates from the Greek for 'siphon' or 'flow through'. The two main symptoms are a great thirst and a need to pass water frequently. The Latin expression *mellitus* was added later. It means 'honeyed', describing the sugary urine that diabetics excrete when the condition is uncontrolled, due to high levels of glucose circulating in the bloodstream.

Types of diabetes

There are two main types of diabetes, which you may have heard being described by different names:

- *Type I* diabetes is insulin-dependent diabetes or IDDM for short, otherwise known as 'juvenile onset diabetes'. Type I is less common than Type II.
- *Type II* is non-insulin-dependent diabetes or NIDDM, sometimes described as 'maturity onset diabetes'.

For ease, this book will use the terms Type I and Type II to describe these two types – which is also how doctors describe them.

Although they are both diabetes, the course of the disease and the way later complications set in are quite different. Patients even look different. Typically, at diagnosis, a Type I diabetic is usually under 30 and thin while a Type II diabetic is over 40 and overweight. Statistically, six per cent of the world's population have Type II diabetes.

The disease

The underlying cause of all diabetes is the body's inability to produce, or efficiently use, the vital hormone insulin which is responsible for converting food into energy.

This happens when insulin-producing cells in the pancreas (the pistol-shaped 'factory' for insulin which lies behind the stomach – see *figure 1*) either stop functioning or cannot produce enough insulin for the body's demands.

Insulin is essential for clearing sugar (the body's energy supply) out of the bloodstream to the body's vital organs and tissues.

Untreated, diabetes can kill, or cause major malfunctions in most of the important body systems, leading to serious complications such as heart and kidney disease, gangrene and blindness.

Type I diabetics are unable to produce *any* insulin. Symptoms usually appear when 70 per cent of the insulin-producing cells in the pancreas are destroyed.

Type II diabetics usually continue to produce *some* insulin, but, for various reasons, the body puts up barriers, or resistance, to it and the insulin cannot work effectively.

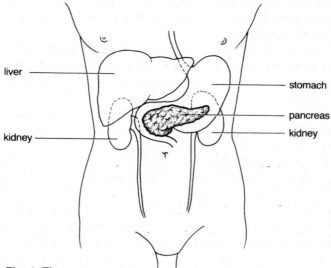

Fig. 1 The pancreas

What does insulin do?

Insulin is a protein made up of 51 amino acids. Not only does it enable glucose to be used by the body as energy, but it also allows glucose to be stored in the liver and muscles, preventing the body from using fat or body protein for energy sources. Insulin also helps the body store fat and repair tissue, so it is vital for health and survival.

Normally, insulin is released into the bloodstream after a meal (see *figure 2*). Its job is to enable the glucose obtained from sweet and starchy foods to reach cells in the nerves and brain which are unable to accept 'fuel' or energy in any form other than glucose.

Insulin is the key to opening the door to the cells, allowing the glucose to enter. When no insulin is produced, the glucose effectively becomes homeless in the bloodstream, denied access to the right body cells and left to float about.

When sugar levels get high enough (we all have our 'renal threshold') the excess glucose spills out into the urine. The kidneys respond to this internal overload by flushing it out of the system (hence the desire to pass urine).

Water is drawn from other body cells for this flushing process – which results in a desperate parched feeling and dehydration.

These twin symptoms are cries for help from a body whose fine-tuning has been seriously thrown out of balance.

Over time, consistently high levels of glucose circulating in the blood start to damage organs, tissues and blood vessels in the body.

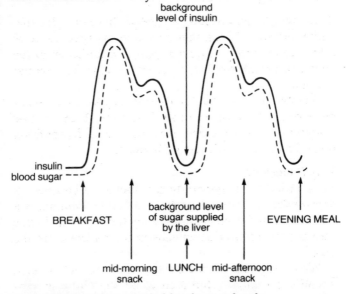

Fig. 2 How insulin controls blood sugar levels
Reproduced with permission from the British Diabetic Association

Type I diabetes

Type I usually surfaces suddenly in children. In Finland, which has the highest diabetes rates of anywhere in the world, and where the condition has increased by 57 per cent in the last 20 years, peak times for diagnosis are ages two, nine, and fourteen in boys and three, five, and eleven in girls.

More evidence is, however, coming to light to show that Type I diabetes can develop later in life, and although adult onset is rare it can in theory affect anyone at any age. Classic symptoms are:

- a frequent need to pass urine
- enormous thirst
- tiredness and irritability
- loss of weight, and a thin body

If the symptoms are left untreated there is a decline, with more weight loss, vomiting, and the appearance of *ketones* in the urine (toxic byproducts resulting from the body's use of fat supplies for energy), eventually leading to coma.

Scientists believe that the disease may take months or even years to manifest itself. But once all the classic symptoms have appeared, it is too late to do anything other than treat the disease with insulin.

Why it happens

Type I diabetes is generally considered to be an *auto-immune disease*. That means the body's own immune system attacks and destroys apparently healthy cells. In this case the insulin-producing cells in the pancreas are the target.

What triggers this hostile action is the subject of much scientific speculation, but it could be something as common as a virus or an environmental toxin.

Summary

In Type I diabetes:

- The majority of cases appear in childhood, with a peak time around puberty.
- Ten per cent of cases have one affected relative already.
- It is more common among Europeans.
- It is most often diagnosed in the summer.
- It is slightly more common among boys than girls.

Type II diabetes

Classically, Type II diabetes affects the over 40s and the overweight, and is by far the most common type of the disease, accounting for between 75 and 90 per cent of all cases.

Diabetes may already be in the family and there is likely to be a slow and insidious decline before the disease takes grip. In America it is estimated that there are at least six million people who are diabetics but don't even know it, because symptoms only appear once the disease is well established.

The descent into the disease can take several years and during this time sufferers may have *impaired glucose tolerance* (higher than normal blood-sugar levels), a condition which can be identified by blood tests. Sufferers often have a lifestyle that involves them sitting around a lot and eating a high fat diet. Men are likely to have pot bellies, and women to have a lot of upper body fat. Symptoms are:

- tiredness
- the need to pass urine often, maybe several times a night

- a craving to drink great quantities of liquid, maybe up to 3½ pints (2 litres) a meal
- blurred vision

Why it happens

Type II diabetics may still produce insulin, but either it is not effective, or not enough is being produced by the insulin factory, the pancreas.

Some 80 per cent of people with Type II diabetes are overweight. Being overweight and inactive encourages insulin resistance, which means the insulin that is produced does not reach the correct receptors in the body cells. Sometimes there may be too few insulin receptors to allow the glucose to enter and be used for fuel.

Type II diabetics may also have impaired or abnormal insulin secretion after meals, leading to high levels of glucose in the bloodstream.

This type of diabetes tends to run in families. This means either there is a genetic link or the seeds of Type II diabetes could be sown as early as the baby's development in the womb (see *Chapter 2*).

Gestational diabetes

This is a third variety of diabetes which affects about 4 per cent of pregnant women and is usually picked up during routine blood tests after the twentieth week of pregnancy.

Why it happens

During pregnancy, blood glucose levels rise in response to pregnancy hormones, and in some women the pancreas cannot keep up with the demands for the extra insulin to keep blood sugar levels in balance.

Women with gestational diabetes often have big babies. The extra glucose circulating in the mother's

blood crosses the placenta to the foetus, which responds
by making extra insulin of its own. The combination of
excess glucose and excess insulin can make the baby fat,
and once born the baby can be at risk of *hypoglycaemia*,
very low blood-sugar levels.

Women who get diabetes in pregnancy may not have
had any symptoms before, and once the baby is born the
symptoms usually disappear.

However, 40 per cent of women who experience gestational diabetes will go on to develop fully fledged diabetes later in life, usually Type II but occasionally Type I.

Unlike the other varieties, there are few obvious
symptoms. But regular antenatal checks would make
sure the tests are done that would detect it.

Maturity Onset Diabetes in the Young (MODY)

This type of diabetes was only identified 20 years ago
and it is still considered rare. MODY carries all the classic
symptoms of Type II diabetes but occurs in young people under the age of 25.

The need for insulin to control the disease is not so
great and in some cases the complications of diabetes
never develop. There is thought to be a strong inherited or
genetic factor in the development of this type of diabetes.

Brittle diabetes

A term sometimes heard, particularly in connection with
diabetes in young people, is 'brittle diabetes'. This is not
a special type of diabetes but a term used to describe
instability in the disease. It means someone – often
teenage girls – undergoing severe highs and lows in
blood glucose levels. Brittle diabetes usually settles
down at maturity.

Other types and causes

Rarely, diabetes can be caused by another disease such as *pancreatitis*, hormonal conditions such as Cushing's disease and *acromegaly* (over-production of growth hormones).

Large amounts of steroids and large doses of certain diuretics can also cause diabetes.

Complications

Before the discovery of insulin in 1921 by two Canadian medical researchers Dr Frederick Banting and medical student Charles Best, 82 per cent of Type I diabetics died within two years of diagnosis. Type II diabetes went largely unrecognized.

It was not until insulin was used to treat diabetics and prolong their life that the long-term complications of the disease were recognized. Insulin was saving diabetics – but it was not preventing the complications.

There are two types of complication:

- conditions that can arise on a day-by-day basis
- long-term effects

Everyday risks

- *Hypoglycaemia* Sometimes known as insulin reaction or insulin shock, this affects diabetics who have to inject insulin or take glucose-lowering drugs to control their disease. It happens when too much insulin circulates in the blood, causing excessively low blood sugar levels. This might be as a result of missing a meal but still having an injection of insulin, or during exercise when blood sugar levels will drop anyway.

Having a 'hypo'

Most diabetics get to know their own warning signals for a
hypo (an attack of hypoglycaemia). Recently there have
been complaints that some of the new types of genetically
created insulin treatments (called human insulin) numb
these sensations, which can be potentially dangerous. There
is more on this in *Chapter 5*. The symptoms might include:

- feeling shaky
- sickness
- hunger
- feeling hot and sticky

There could be mood swings, irritability, and irrationality,
coupled with a tingling sensation around the mouth, a lack of
concentration and blurred vision.

   The treatment is to eat something sugary like a couple of
biscuits, to balance out the levels of glucose and insulin in
the bloodstream.

- *Hyperglycaemia* This means there is too much sugar
  circulating and not enough insulin and may be the
  first sign of out of control diabetes.
- *Ketoacidosis* Stress can be a factor in this potentially
  fatal complication of diabetes, in which the body is
  slowly poisoned by internal toxins. Prolonged stress
  can cause blood sugar levels to rise rapidly. When the
  body requires energy but cannot get it from glucose
  circulating in the blood, the brain calls on the liver to
  deliver extra supplies. More glucose pours into the
  bloodstream, raising blood sugar levels even higher.
  But all to no avail. Without insulin none of this essential glucose can get to the cells. The brain then calls on
  another energy source – fat. This offers an immediate
  answer, because when fat is burned energy is released.
  But the 'down' side is that toxic acids called *ketones* are
  also produced as a byproduct. Too many cause

ketoacidosis. The first symptoms are nausea, followed by the two classic symptoms of thirst and excessive urination as the body once again desperately tries to flush out the toxins. Dehydration can follow, then abdominal pain, drowsiness and rapid breathing. The eventual outcome is *diabetic coma* and if the condition is not treated immediately in hospital, by restoring hydration and insulin levels, it can result in death.

- *Blurry vision*   If glucose levels are running high, the lens of the eye can become distorted, causing blurred vision. Once levels are lowered, the blurred vision usually clears up.

Long-term complications

Microvascular disease, affecting the small blood vessels in the body, and macrovascular disease, affecting the large, are the two key long-term complications of diabetes. High or uncontrolled blood glucose levels can:

- thicken the lining of small blood vessels, called capillaries, making them leak, or unable to supply nutrients to tissues
- cause the free-floating, or unused, glucose to stick to proteins in the body, causing stiff hands and joints
- damage and block nerve pathways
- cause arteries to fur up

Microvascular disease
Microvascular disease, damage to small blood vessels or capillaries, can cause the following:

Eye problems
If you have diabetes, it is important to have eye tests regularly, as high glucose levels in the blood can affect all parts of the eye, and long periods of uncontrolled diabetes can lead to blurred vision and eventually to blindness.

In Europe, 46 per cent of Type I diabetics experience some damage to the retina. In Britain *diabetic retinopathy* is the single most common cause of blindness among adults between the ages of 55 and 64.

High glucose levels can create blockages in the small blood vessels in the *retina*, the light-sensitive part of the back of the eye which sends pictures of what we see along the optic nerve to the brain. To make up for this blockage other vessels open up or dilate, and the trouble begins when these enlarged vessels begin to leak blood.

In the case of *proliferative retinopathy* new blood vessels form on the surface of the retina. If they leak into the centre of the retina, called the *macula*, vision can become blurred or, in the worst cases, lost completely. An eye-specialist can treat retinopathy by laser surgery.

Note It is dangerous to exercise if you are suffering from this condition. It could pose a serious threat to your vision.

Eye problems and diabetes

- At diagnosis 25 per cent of patients with Type II diabetes have already suffered changes to the blood vessels in the retina.
- Chronic glaucoma and cataracts are more common in people with diabetes.
- Two per cent of diabetics go blind because of diabetic retinopathy.

Kidney damage
Diabetes is the second most common cause of kidney damage – *nephropathy* – for patients who need dialysis or transplantation.

It happens when small blood vessels in the kidneys become thickened, and cannot perform their job of filtering waste products out of the blood into the urine. As it worsens, the kidney function deteriorates and, in the end-stage, kidney transplant is the only solution.

Nerve damage

High or uncontrolled blood glucose can create a short-circuiting effect on the complex web which makes up the nervous system.

The coating of a fatty substance which protects the nerves can be damaged and the small blood vessels feeding the nerves can become blocked, leading to loss of sensation and numbness.

You may get to hear about a condition called *peripheral neuropathy*, because it is the most common type of nerve damage, generally affecting the feet, legs, arms and hands.

This can cause tingling in the affected areas, and eventually numbness, so injuries are more difficult to detect, leading to infections which become hard to treat. In the worst cases it can result in gangrene and amputation. Feet are most commonly affected, so it is wise to check them routinely.

Autonomic neuropathy is the damage to nerves serving the heart and blood vessels and other internal organs that can affect blood pressure.

Sexual problems

Impotence is the most common sexual complication. It strikes when the nerves carrying the signals to the blood vessels needed for an erection become damaged by diabetes. Although the mind is willing, the body cannot function. There are devices that can help men with impotence, so seek guidance from your family doctor. Another problem is *retrograde ejaculation* – being unable to ejaculate despite having an orgasm.

In women, the nerve damage caused by diabetes can affect sexual performance, causing difficulties with lubrication and orgasm.

Particular problems for women

In September 1994 the *Journal of the American Dietetic Association* published a study on why diabetes should be considered a priority healthcare issue for women.

There are 3.3 million American women diagnosed with diabetes and the report pointed out that 60 per cent of all new cases are diagnosed in women.

It concluded that:

- Type I diabetics have more problems in pregnancy.
- Twice as many women die from diabetes and related illnesses as from breast cancer.
- Female diabetics are more at risk from eating disorders and from endometrial cancer.

Macrovascular disease
Macrovascular disease, damage to large blood vessels, can cause the following:

Heart disease
Male diabetics run three times the risk of developing cardiovascular disease, and pre-menopausal diabetic women run four times the risk.

Hardening of the arteries
Hardening of the arteries (*arteriosclerosis* or *atherosclerosis*) occurs in almost everyone as they age, whether they are diabetic or not. It is caused by fatty deposits building up and hardening in the arteries so they become 'furred up' and narrowed.

Sometimes this condition is accelerated in diabetics. This can lead to higher risks of heart attacks, stroke and poor circulation.

High blood pressure
High blood pressure, or *hypertension*, is a common complication and two-thirds of adults with diabetes have hypertension.

Syndrome X

A cluster of conditions associated with diabetes make up this so-called Syndrome X, or *Reaven's Syndrome*:

- raised levels of fats (*lipids*) in the blood
- high blood pressure
- layers of fat in the abdominal region (otherwise known as a 'pot belly')
- insulin resistance, a condition known as *hyperinsulinaemia*

How complications differ for Type I and Type II diabetes

- Microvascular disease is more of a problem for Type I diabetics, while Type II diabetics tend to succumb to macrovascular complications.
- Between 30 and 50 per cent of Type I diabetics will develop diabetic kidney disease, while only a fraction of Type IIs will suffer this complication.
- Nearly 40 per cent of Type II diabetics have some form of eye damage when they are diagnosed, while Type Is might not develop any eye complications for some years after diagnosis. (A European multi-centre study of complications found an incidence of eye complications in Type Is of just 7 per cent within five years of diagnosis – but this rose steeply after that and after 20 years it averages 82 per cent.)

Can the risk of complications be reduced?

The answer is yes. A major American trial called the Diabetes Control and Complications Trial (DCCT) which was carried out in 29 centres and involved 1,441 Type I diabetics has conclusively shown that tight blood glucose control – that is, keeping blood sugar levels to within a normal range – reduces the risks of complications by as much as 60 per cent.

However, there are some down sides to tight control, or *intensive therapy* as it is otherwise known. It can cause weight gain and more 'hypos' (episodes of severe low blood glucose).

Intensive therapy means:

- frequent self-monitoring of blood glucose
- careful attention to diet and exercise

It may not be suitable for:

- small children
- the elderly
- pregnant women
- those with a history of low sugar reactions

A similar trial, called the UK Prospective Diabetes Study (UKPDS), is currently investigating whether similar control in Type II diabetics has the same beneficial effect – that is, preventing or delaying complications. The UK trial is looking at the effect of diet, diet and tablet treatment, and insulin treatment.

Type II diabetics can use intensive therapy to control their diabetes – but blood sugar monitoring may not have to be done quite so frequently. If you are managing your diabetes by diet alone, once a week could be enough. If you take tablets, once a day would probably be sufficient.

Can diabetes be cured?

No. Once diabetes is diagnosed there is no going back. The only cure is a pancreatic transplant, but this is a last and rare resort and only considered in conjunction with a kidney transplant. There have been some success stories with these sort of operations, and patients have been able to give up insulin – only to replace it with strong anti-rejection drugs.

Summary

- Once diagnosed, Type I diabetics face a lifetime of medication to replace the insulin they are incapable of producing. The amount of insulin required depends on how well they are able to encourage their body's uptake, and natural therapies can stimulate this action.
- If you are a Type II diabetic you will not be able to cure your diabetes, but you do have the power, without recourse to tablets or injections in some cases, to control it – rather than allowing the disease to control you.
- All diabetics should be able to live a normal and long life, without pain and suffering. But it takes self-discipline and regular monitoring.
- The later, serious complications of the disease *can* be delayed or prevented, if you wise up to the need to keep your diabetes under control.

This book aims to empower diabetics and their family and friends to find new ways of controlling their diabetes, so that they can live a normal and full life, with the fear of complications greatly reduced.

But before you can begin to make changes you need to understand a little more about the mechanics of the disease, who is at risk, and why.

CHAPTER 2

Triggers and causes
of diabetes

What they are and how they affect us

Diabetes can strike at random so, technically, we are all at risk of this disease of the Western world. No one has identified a single cause for diabetes, but there are plenty of theories.

It is generally accepted that both main types of diabetes are deeply rooted in genetics – that is, the causes are born with us. So those most at risk are those born with a *genetic susceptibility* to the disease. With Type I diabetes there are thought to be at least nine genes involved, so this is a very complex area of debate and study.

In February 1995 Dr Simon Bennett of the UK Welcome Trust Centre for Human Genetics in Oxford, England, announced his discovery of a specific DNA defect within the insulin gene in the part which 'controls' how much insulin is produced. Although there are many genes that apparently predispose towards diabetes this is only the second flaw, or mutation, to be identified.

The mutation occurs more often in people with Type I diabetes. The discovery is another part of the jigsaw which will all come together one day in the future to provide the answer to the cause of diabetes.

The gene theory might help explain the diabetes 'hot spots' around the world. But genetics cannot explain why, among sets of identical twins, only about a third are *both* affected. Most doctors believe there have to be other, probably environmental, influences.

Being genetically susceptible does not always mean that you will develop diabetes. There has to be a trigger, something which sparks the disease off.

The trigger which starts the destruction of insulin-producing cells in the pancreas, or stops insulin reaching the correct cells, could be one of many things or a combination of several.

Among the current popular theories are:

For Type I diabetes
- a virus
- protein in cow's milk
- environmental toxins
- stress
- where you live

For Type II diabetes
- obesity and over-eating, plus lack of exercise
- culture and lifestyle
- age
- continuously raised blood sugar levels
- stress
- low birthweight, or malnutrition in the womb

Type I diabetes triggers

A *virus*

Type I diabetes is most often diagnosed in the spring, autumn and winter, and often after a child has been ill with a virus. The link between viruses and Type I diabetes was made as long ago as the 1800s, following reports of diabetes developing after episodes of infectious disease.

Amongst common viruses suspected are the mumps virus (which can cause acute pancreatitis and sometimes hyperglycaemia), rubella or the 'German measles' virus (40 per cent of babies who contract rubella in the womb develop diabetes later in life), cytomegalovirus, echovirus, herpes, polio, tick-borne encephalitis, infectious hepatitis, and the Coxsackie B viruses that cause diarrhoeal illnesses.

Coxsackie B-type viruses bear a remarkable molecular similarity to the beta cells in the pancreas (which produce insulin) and the theory is that the virus somehow fools the body's auto-immune system into attacking the insulin-producing cells in the pancreas, believing them to be 'hostile'.

Cow's milk

The protein in cow's milk is a prime suspect as a trigger for Type I diabetes. The development of Type I diabetes is up to 50 per cent higher among children who are bottle-fed. Researchers have discovered that an immune response to the protein can develop in genetically susceptible children.

There are other clues. Finland, with the highest incidence of Type I diabetes to be found anywhere, also leads the world in milk consumption. Also, the people of Western Samoa had no known cases of Type I diabetes until they emigrated to New Zealand and drank cow's milk for the first time.

In an attempt to find out more, a major ten-year study is under way in Canada and Finland, following the progress of 2,000 newborn babies and their drinking of cow's milk during the first nine months of their life.

What is certain is that prolonged breast-feeding gives some protection against the disease.

Environmental toxins

Food additives, rat poison, highly refined food, ultraviolet radiation from the sun, even smoked foods and cassava have all been considered as potential triggers at some time.

Stress
Stress might be a contributory factor and speed the process of cell destruction in some susceptible people (see *chapter 8* for more details).

Where you live
The highest rates of diabetes are to be found across Europe. The World Health Organization's project for Childhood Diabetes (DIAMOND), which examined data from over 40 countries, reported a clear difference in the incidence of diabetes between the northern and southern hemispheres. Below the equator, Type I diabetes is relatively rare (apart from Australia and New Zealand), although it may be that statistics are not so well kept in these countries, or that diabetes is not routinely picked up.

Above the equator, this form of diabetes is a common and escalating disease, with the rates rising across Europe. In Finland, the country with the highest rate of all for diabetes, the figures are continuing to climb at alarming rates. A child in Finland is 50 times more likely to develop diabetes than a child in Korea or China and 10 times more likely to develop the disease than a child in Greece.

There are even regional differences within one area. In the British Isles, for example, Scotland has twice as high an incidence of Type I diabetes as the Republic of Ireland.

Researchers have evidence of abrupt increases from time to time. They are not technically 'epidemics' because these hiccups in the statistics are not necessarily followed by falls in the number of people affected, and it may have something to do with the genetic pool widening: for example, more women with Type I diabetes survive to have children of their own.

Type II diabetes triggers

Obesity and lack of exercise
Some 80 per cent of Type II diabetics are overweight, and being fat encourages insulin resistance. Obesity is defined as an 'abundance of fat tissue' – people who weigh 20 per cent above their 'ideal body weight' are technically obese.

An accurate way to assess how overweight you are is to calculate your Body Mass Index (BMI), which is worked out by your weight in kilograms divided by height in metres squared. Obesity is defined as a BMI above 30.

Type II diabetes is strongly linked to a high fat diet. Taking up exercise encourages the body to use insulin more effectively and for some diabetics this may be the only form of natural treatment required to manage the disease successfully.

Researchers from the American Dietetic Association have shown that even moderate weight loss can mean a 20 to 75 per cent reduction in risk factors for Type II diabetes as well as high blood pressure and heart disease.

The researchers discovered that the most critical pounds lost are the first ones and that the key is to lose fat while increasing the percentage of lean tissue. That means exercise.

Culture and lifestyle
People who move and settle in other countries develop Type II diabetes more often than the local population. For example, there is a higher incidence of diabetes among the Asian community in Britain and the Hispanic population in America.

Becoming physically lazy and changing to a higher-fat Western-style diet are leading factors in the theory that a change in lifestyle and culture can trigger Type II diabetes.

The idea that malnutrition in early life might trigger diabetes in later life is borne out by the development of diabetes amongst communities which move from countries where there is too little food to areas where people enjoy too much food. Ethiopian Jews who have moved to Israel, for example, have developed a high rate of diabetes.

Poor nutrition in the womb or as a baby may, somehow, affect the function and structure of the insulin-producing cells in the pancreas and may change the tissues which respond to insulin. It is generally accepted that by the time a baby is a year old, half of its adult beta cells (see *page 29*) will already be present. Influences at this stage of development could well affect the size and structure of the pancreas later.

Malnutrition in the womb is not confined to developing countries. Babies in the West can experience this too if, for example, there is a malfunction in the way the placenta passes nutrition to the growing baby.

Alternatively, it might be that the correct nutrients are not present in the pregnant mother's diet before conception, at the time of conception, or during the nine months of pregnancy.

'It used to be thought that the whole pattern of your life was set at the moment of conception, but it could be that what happens to you in the next nine months actually moulds you', explains Professor David Barker, director of the Medical Research Council's environmental epidemiology unit at the University of Southampton in Britain.

Although he is convinced of the impact of early nutrition on our lives he agrees that other factors such as being overweight, ageing, and physical inactivity also play a part in the timing of the onset of diabetes.

Age

The older we get, the more at risk we are of Type II diabetes. The over 60s are four times more likely to contract Type II diabetes than the general population. It is linked to reduced physical activity, and a natural decrease in insulin activity.

Raised blood sugar levels

More of a warning bell than a trigger, this symptomless condition is technically called *impaired glucose tolerance* (IGT), and can indicate a decline towards diabetes.

However, not everyone with IGT will go on to develop diabetes. There is a test, which takes two hours to complete, to assess blood glucose levels accurately. If you are considered at risk, safe and natural techniques for lowering your glucose levels will do no harm and might actually do a lot of good.

Stress

It has been known for a long time that blood glucose levels rise when we are under stress, feeling sad, worried or frustrated. As with Type I diabetes, stress may be a contributory factor rather than a complete trigger.

Low birthweight

Professor Barker has studied links between low birthweight and the development of Type II diabetes later in life. In his book *Mothers, Babies and Disease in Later Life,* he says five studies have shown that men and women with low birthweight have increased rates of Type II diabetes and impaired glucose tolerance.

He says: 'People who were thin at birth, having a low muscle bulk, tend to become insulin resistant and develop Syndrome X – diabetes, hypertension, and raised plasma triglycerides [a type of fat in the blood].'

Should we all be screened for diabetes?

At present no country has a screening programme, mainly because it is a costly exercise. Also, because there are currently no proven conventional remedies to halt the onset of the disease, screening is not considered ethical.

National screening will come about if scientists find an acceptable way of stopping diabetes in the pre-diabetic phase. Professor Edwin Gale and researchers at St Bartholomew's Hospital in London are refining 'prediction testing' for Type I diabetes in the under fives, using a combination of markers and an antibody test in preparation for this.

Should I get tested?

Like everything else to do with diabetes, it is up to you to take matters into your own hands. You have to decide whether you are at risk, and if so what you plan to do about it.

Blood glucose tests can be organized through family doctors just like blood cholesterol checks. If you do have raised blood glucose levels your doctor will not be able to suggest any formal measures, but there are a number of actions you can take to help yourself (or ask others to help you with) and these are explained in more detail in *Chapter 4* and later in the book. You could also ask your doctor for regular tests to see whether there is any noticeable change in the blood sugar levels.

Type II diabetes and a susceptibility to high blood-glucose levels can strike at random, but in many cases there is a genetic link. Someone in the family might already have the disease.

Testing for diabetes

Testing the level of glucose in the blood gives a clear indication of whether insulin production is normal. The World Health Organization has laid down a set of guidelines for an oral glucose-tolerance blood test which can diagnose:

- normal blood sugar levels
- impaired glucose tolerance
- diabetes

The test is explained in greater detail in *Chapter 5*.

Once diagnosed as a diabetic you will have to come to terms with doing your own daily blood sugar tests. Most diabetics use speedy finger prick devices which can give you a result within a matter of seconds (see *figure 3*).

The finger prick test is not a definitive diagnostic test but simply an aid to managing diabetes. It measures blood glucose levels from the capillaries and not a main vein where concentrations of glucose could be higher.

Another way of testing for diabetes is testing for glucose in the urine. This can give an indication of diabetes, but cannot be used to diagnose it.

Borderline diabetes

A high proportion of people with impaired glucose tolerance (IGT) go on to develop diabetes. This is a condition in which blood glucose levels are higher than normal, but are not critical enough for any treatment.

Those at risk from developing diabetes (you may have IGT and have a relative in the family with diabetes) could do a lot to help themselves during this phase, and, with the proper advice, even delay the establishment of the disease.

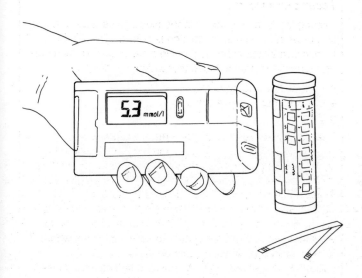

Fig. 3 A typical blood glucose monitoring kit

Diet and exercise are key treatments, and other gentle forms of therapy such as relaxation and yoga have been found to help reduce blood glucose levels. But remember, not everyone who has this condition will go on to develop diabetes. The condition might last for years, or correct itself, with blood glucose levels returning to normal.

The pancreas

The pancreas is a gland and a hormone-producing 'factory'. Not only does it make and control production and output of insulin, but it is also busy storing and releasing other hormones such as *glucagon* which has the opposite effect of insulin – it raises the blood sugar levels. Another part of the pancreas also makes digestive juices which are mixed with food when it leaves the stomach.

Insulin production in the pancreas is looked after by *beta cells* in the part known as 'the islets of Langerhans' (after the doctor who discovered them). Beta cells are the clusters of cells in the pancreas responsible for stimulating the release of insulin. Like brain cells, beta cells are 'electrically excitable' and respond to glucose in the bloodstream.

Glucagon production is looked after by *alpha cells* found clustered in these same islets, or pools of cells. Together these islets make up about 1 per cent of the pancreas.

Latest research

The international search for the genes responsible for diabetes is providing new information about who is at risk from diabetes. In 1994 two new genes were identified, one to chromosome 6 and the other to chromosome 11. Dr John Todd of Oxford University, one of the team which made the discovery, believes there could between 9 and 12 genes involved.

To find the genes Dr Todd and a team of medical researchers recruited 300 families in Britain and America in which two children have insulin dependent diabetes but their parents do not. The logic behind this approach is that if two children are sufferers, and neither parent is, the children must have inherited certain gene combinations that make them susceptible to the disease.

Approximately 90 per cent of new cases of Type I diabetes strike in families with no immediate history of diabetes and how families cope when this happens is described in the next chapter.

CHAPTER 3

Children and diabetes

The problems and the solutions

Most cases of Type I or insulin dependent diabetes are diagnosed in childhood, either in infancy, or the teen years.

The natural way with diabetes and children is to encourage your child to become fully involved in his or her diabetes care, to encourage independence at an early age, and to keep lines of communication open, especially during difficult teen years.

Bringing up a child with diabetes can mean negotiating a series of minefields. The family with a diabetic child might have a toddler who won't eat, a school age child who feels different to his or her friends, and a teenager who rebels and refuses insulin, or suffers from an eating disorder. This is all normal, natural, and part of growing up with a diabetic child.

The first task for parents is coming to terms with the fact that their child has been diagnosed with a life-long incurable illness. Parents speak of feelings of devastation and guilt, and of fears for the future.

Lorrayne, mother of a four-year-old boy, Adam, diagnosed at three, is an example: 'I had suspected it was diabetes. Adam used to get so thirsty he would wake up in the morning and ask for grapefruit juice, milk, water, all at once. He was even slurping the bath water.

'When I did get him to the doctors, a urine test showed his glucose level was astronomically high and he was admitted to hospital the same day, where we stayed for a week. I could have kicked myself for not acting more quickly.'

Who is most at risk

- If a child has a mother, father, brother or sister with Type I diabetes then he or she is 20 times more at risk from the disease than the rest of the population.
- Children have a higher risk of inheriting diabetes through their father's genes than through their mother's genes.
- The peak age for diagnosing Type I diabetes in children is 12.
- Puberty is a time when the body is undergoing all sorts of hormonal changes and a susceptibility to the disease by way of the genes may be triggered by these major hormonal fluctuations.

Symptoms to watch for are:

- constantly asking for drinks
- passing a lot of urine (one mother described how her two-year-old daughter continually filled her potty 'to the brim')
- mood swings – irritability and wingeing
- lethargy and tiredness
- weight loss

Toddler years

The key to coping with a diabetic child is flexibility, and managing the disease without passing on your own fears and worries.

Many parents will agree that it is not the insulin injections which prove to be difficult to manage, it is the finger prick blood testing that is most hated by the child – because it hurts more!

When your child is first diagnosed, expect to be admitted to hospital with him or her for between three and ten days. Use this time wisely, to learn all you can about diabetes and what it means for the future, and to get information and help.

You will be taught how to give injections and take blood tests. Choose, with your child's help, a place for the injection on the leg, the buttocks, arm or tummy.

You will be confronted with a whole new world of regular meal times and injections. A child's insulin requirements are usually assessed by weight, but at first it will be a matter of trial and error. There may be plenty of blood glucose testing and monitoring before your child's condition stabilizes. Expect to be asked back to see a specialist every three months. Children grow rapidly, so insulin requirements change rapidly also.

At home, make injection times as pleasant as possible. Relax, choose a comfy place to sit, distract a small child with a toy or book, TV or video. Be kind but firm; a child should never be able to bargain his or her way out of an injection.

How to inject a toddler
Carefully pinch up a fold of skin, insert the needle and slowly release the insulin. Massaging the site will help the insulin to be absorbed more quickly. Give lots of praise, and encouragement. Try to involve your child as much as possible by allowing him or her to get out 'the equipment' or to choose where the injection will be given today.

At first, injecting your child may seem strange and difficult. One mother of an 18-month-old described the first time she injected her son at home alone as the 'most frightening experience of my life'.

Another, on injecting her two-year-old for the first

time, said: 'I became quite detached; I switched off. It was almost as if I could not bear to think what I was doing to my own flesh and blood – yet it still had to be done. This was my way of coping.

'My husband could not stand needles before Jack was diagnosed. But he overcame that, and was determined that he would do it. He learnt how to in hospital, and now gives them quite happily at home.'

In the early years diabetes is much easier for a young child to accept. It simply becomes part of life.

Barbara's story

Barbara Elster formed the first national support network for parents of diabetic children in Britain. It has proved to be a lifeline for many families confronting the disease for the first time.

She believes involving the whole family is vital to ensure other children in the family don't feel left out. When her son Bradley was diagnosed she had three daughters aged four, six and eight. They all grew up knowing, and later understanding, about their brother's disease.

Barbara says one of the most enduring memories of childhood with Bradley was carting what became known as 'the bag' around with them on any family days out. This contained supplies for every possible situation: phials of insulin and syringes and sugary drinks and biscuits (for hypos).

'My son is now 27 and a film cameraman. He still carries a bag around with him wherever he goes in the world', she says.

Toddlers and eating

One of the biggest worries facing parents of toddlers is what happens when a child won't eat or goes through a normal period of faddy eating.

- Adopt a snack routine. Don't expect a young child to stick to three large meals a day like an adult. If your child won't eat, offer plenty to drink – he will eventually get hungry.
- Don't demand he sits down to eat. Remain flexible and offer healthy snacks like a slice of wholemeal bread to chew on as he plays in the garden.
- Accept that blood glucose levels will inevitably fluctuate, as a child's daily life is unpredictable.

School years

Parents have far less control over their child's diabetes once he or she is off to school. It is the start of your child growing up, and becoming more independent, and this is the next hurdle to confront.

Get as much support as you can from your specialist diabetic nurse or natural therapist; talk to the school; explain to the teachers. Let everyone know that your child can't be punished by having a late lunch or missing a vital snack at break time.

Children don't need to be made to feel different – they can eat a mid-morning snack at playtime, just like all the other children.

Teachers should know what to do in the event of a hypo. You should ensure your child has a supply of biscuits or sugary drinks if his blood sugar levels fall at school.

Encourage independence by:

- using positive reinforcement – rewarding good actions instead of nagging about contrary behaviour

- keeping a chart that shows a child what he or she should be doing each day and reward with stars. Your child can cash them in for a special 'prize' or gift.
- not being tempted to punish for lapses – focus on getting it right tomorrow
- avoiding too much emphasis on denial or saying 'no'
- boosting self-esteem through encouraging self-care

Teen years

Adolescence can cause some of the biggest headaches in any family. St Bartholomew's Hospital in London has opened one of the first adolescent clinics specifically for diabetic teenagers who are in the process of taking over their diabetes management from their parents.

Teenagers often seem incapable of following their self-care routines, have mood swings, are grumpy and distant. This is normal and will often have more to do with hormonal changes that no one can control.

The way the family responds can be vital at this stage. An over-protective or nagging parent will produce an overly dependent or rebellious child. Other tips are:

- Don't become too rigid over daily routine. A teenager will rebel more, or experiment by stopping injections, if his or her parents adopt too rigid an approach.
- Avoid battles over food. Diabetic teenage girls are more prone to *anorexia nervosa* (the so-called 'slimmer's disease') and other eating disorders than those in the general population.
- Support your child's wish to take control.
- Keep lines of communication open rather than get involved in a battle of wills. Involve a third party.

The effect of stress on teenagers
In teenage years, hormones will be running rampant and stress levels, due to exams and the normal problems an

adolescent faces forging an individual personality can also affect glucose control. Your growing child may want to try some of the relaxation therapies mentioned later in the book.

If your child is ill

- Ensure plenty of drinks are offered.
- Don't stop the insulin injections.
- Monitor blood glucose levels and act accordingly.
- If your child is being sick, continue with drinks or herbal teas sweetened with honey.
- Try to tempt your child with a digestive biscuit if he or she can't manage a full meal.

Latest research

Two major studies which began in 1994 promise major developments in the prevention of diabetes in both children and adults – but not until after the year 2000.

The Nicotinamide Trial

Nicotinamide is a B group vitamin, and small amounts are found in a normal healthy diet. Early studies have shown that high doses can protect the insulin-producing beta cells in the pancreas from attack by the body's immune system.

A total of 24 European countries, with Canada and America, have now joined together to take part in the European Nicotinamide Diabetes Intervention Trial (ENDIT).

Over 500 relatives of Type I diabetics, aged between 5 and 40, and considered to be at risk of developing diabetes over the next 10 years, are being recruited into the trial and offered nicotinamide. A blood test shows whether the antibodies which attack insulin-producing cells are forming in the blood.

Jill's story

Jill's son Michael was diagnosed as an insulin dependent diabetic at three. 'Michael was always drinking a lot and never put on much weight, but we did not think it odd at first: both my husband and I are quite small.

'At the end of August Michael had an ear and throat infection after which he ended up begging for drinks. He would then wee a lot, which we put down to all his drinking.

'I gave him milk, fruit drinks, squash, but it became excessive. We were due to go on holiday to Cyprus when we weighed Michael and found he had lost two pounds [one kilogram] in weight. I took him to the doctor's surgery where they ran a urine test: the strip turned dark blue, which meant he had very high levels of sugar in his urine.

'Within the next two hours we were in hospital and Type I diabetes was diagnosed. I felt ghastly, upset and desperate but you have to just get on and cope.'

Six months after diagnosis the family is coming to terms with Michael's diabetes: 'In a way it's easier being diagnosed earlier rather than later as he will know nothing else. We are more relaxed, and he even goes to parties where he eats what he wants, and we manage to work round it.

'We even managed to have that holiday in Cyprus. I took everything we needed with us, including lots of low sugar drinks.'

You are at risk from Type I diabetes over the next ten years if you:

- have a first degree relative with Type I diabetes
- have a strong positive antibody test
- are under 40

Note The ENDIT trial is using large amounts of highly purified nicotinamide. Nicotinamide supplements are available from healthfood stores but they are nothing like as pure and should not be taken in such large amounts.

Natural food sources of nicotinamide are yeast, lean meat, liver and chicken with lesser amounts in milk, canned salmon and leafy green vegetables.

The NIH Insulin Trial

In 1995 ten centres in America began a seven-year trial to find out whether 'immunizing' against the earliest signs of Type I diabetes will prevent it from developing.

The immunization involves twice daily injections of insulin which, in small-scale studies, have been shown to have a preventive effect.

The point of giving insulin *before* it is needed is that if it can delay the onset of Type I diabetes, then the life-threatening complications of the disease can also be delayed, and may be prevented.

Summary

Teaching self-reliance is an important part of helping children come to terms with their diabetes. A diagnosis of diabetes calls for the development of a great deal of self-discipline, and one bonus for some parents is that often children with diabetes develop a remarkable maturity as a result of this responsibility.

The next chapter will look at the various self-help methods for diabetics of all ages.

CHAPTER 4

How to help yourself

Self-help techniques for you and your family

'The sufferer is not disabled mentally or morally. His powers of thinking and acting are unimpaired. By the exercise of will and intelligence he is able to keep well', said the writer H G Wells in a letter, published in *The Times* of London in 1934, with which he founded the British Diabetic Association.

Wells is not the only famous person to have suffered or suffer from diabetes. Beethoven, the jazz musician Dizzy Gillespie, Stan Laurel (of Laurel and Hardy), the actress Mary Tyler Moore and British singer and comic actor Sir Harry Secombe are just some of the high achievers who have also been diabetic. The point is that none of them let diabetes stand in the way of doing what they wanted. They did it anyway.

The key to self-help in diabetes is deciding that you really do want to make changes to improve your lifestyle and health, and to reap the benefits in future years. There are several natural methods which have been shown to have the potential to change the course of your diabetes. They all come under the headings of:

- diet
- exercise
- stress management

Specialist diabetic nurses say that urging their patients

to lose weight and watch what they eat is the hardest challenge they face on a day-to-day basis.

Changing eating habits and routines from 'bad' to 'good', introducing new weight loss programmes or exercise when you are middle-aged and set in your ways, is a difficult prospect, but this is the challenge that confronts most Type II diabetics. It takes will-power and a certain amount of motivation, even if you know that what happens today could affect your health in future years.

Diet

There are two approaches to diet for diabetics:

- dieting (to lose weight)
- diet, meaning nutrition, or daily intake of food (which will be discussed in greater detail in *Chapter 9*)

For Type II diabetics being overweight can prevent insulin from actively working in the body, so aiming for your 'correct weight for height' will not only improve your diabetic control, but will also delay some of the complications (see *figure 4*).

The 'official' advice for diabetics is to stick to a healthy, natural diet with plenty of fresh fruit and veg-etables, lean meats and little saturated fat.

A high carbohydrate diet is often recommended for diabetics – but there is some debate over whether this is now the best approach. Researchers are coming round to the view that a diet rich in monounsaturated fat may be preferable to a high carbohydrate diet because of its abil-ity both to lower glucose levels and maintain healthy levels of 'good' *lipids* (blood fats) in the bloodstream, such as high density lipoprotein (HDL) cholesterol.

Generally speaking, it is best to avoid any very low calorie diets incorporating milkshakes or powders as they can lead to loss of vital trace elements and minerals.

Fifty years ago diabetics were put on starvation rations as a form of treatment. Today the advice is to choose foods from across the range, in moderation.

Losing weight safely and effectively is a matter of burning up more energy (calories) than you take in. Energy comes mostly from what we eat and drink (and from the air we breathe) so the only effective way to lose weight is to eat less.

A good weight loss programme is one which is as natural as possible, makes sure you lose weight gradually,

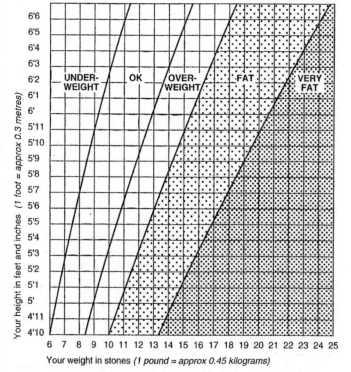

Fig. 4 Ideal weight-to-height chart

but regularly, and does not see the weight go back on when you stop.

Diabetics need to eat three meals a day including breakfast and, like everyone else, to eat a wide variety of foods for maximum health benefits.

An American report, the *Nutritional Principles for the Management of Diabetes and Related Complications*, published in 1994, says even a moderate calorie restriction (of between 250 and 500 calories a day) can have an impact on Type II diabetics.

To lose weight, the secret is to avoid foods full of saturated fat and sugar (which should be largely excluded from a diabetic diet in any case) and only eat enough to meet 70 per cent of your daily energy requirements. *For maximum effect it is important to diet and exercise together.*

Diabetics are more at risk of raised levels of 'bad' low density lipoprotein (LDL) cholesterol and other fats in the bloodstream which considerably increase the risk of heart disease. But remember, not all fats are bad. *Saturated fat* is thought to be the main 'baddie'. Found in animal foods like red meat and dairy products, it has also been linked to high blood cholesterol.

To cut down on saturated fat:

- Eat lean cuts of meat or remove all extra fat.
- Eat more fish and poultry (though diabetics should steer clear of oily fish such as mackerel: there is evidence that oily fish – containing omega-6 oils – can raise blood glucose levels, even though another sort, the omega-3 oils, help lower cholesterol levels).
- Use diet spread rather than butter.
- Drink low fat or skimmed milk.
- Limit your number of eggs to three or four a week.
- Avoid pork sausages, pork pies, hamburgers, French fries (chips), full fat milk, cream cakes, cheddar cheese.

Two other forms of fats, *monounsaturated* and *polyunsaturated*, are good for everyone but there is evidence they are particularly good for diabetics.

Monounsaturated fat is the most beneficial for diabetics (see *Chapter 9*) but only buy the cold-pressed extra virgin type of oil, as olive oil extracted using heat is changed and may become harmful.

Polyunsaturated fat is also good for you in moderate amounts. It is found in vegetable oil, such as corn and sunflower oil.

The other food to beware of is *sugar*. Sugar turns to body fat if it is not burned up as energy. Too much sugar in the diet can lead to chromium deficiency, an important trace element for diabetics.

Unless you are a Type I diabetic and need an emergency supply of wholemeal biscuits or small chocolate bars, avoid the temptation of buying any biscuits and chocolate. If it is not in the cupboard you can't eat it.

The way to healthy eating

- Eat regularly. Have three meals a day including breakfast.
- Eat a wide variety of foods.
- Eat plenty of foods rich in starch and fibre.
- Eat more fruit and vegetables.
- Avoid foods containing large amounts of saturated fat and sugar.
- Replace saturated fats with monounsaturated fats.
- Eat the right amount to maintain a healthy weight.

It is best to try to ensure you get adequate nutrients from eating fresh, wholesome, preferably organic food, rather than just from vitamin and mineral supplements. There is evidence that excessive levels of some vitamins (such as vitamin C) could, in some cases, be harmful for diabetics – even though they may be perfectly safe for others. If you need to lose weight, aim to lose no more than 1–2 pounds (½–1 kilograms) a week.

Beware also of *salt* (sodium chloride). Too much can lead to high blood pressure, particularly in diabetics. Try using herbs and spices instead or lemon juice on vegetables.

Diet plan

The following should form part of a healthy diet plan.

- *Starchy foods*. These should form a main part of meals and snacks. They are filling, a good source of nutrition, and cheap. They are also a good source of fibre. Choose from wholemeal bread, pitta bread, wholegrain crispbread, wholegrain cereal (without added salt or sugar), unsweetened porridge, muesli (unsweetened), boiled and baked potatoes, boiled rice, pasta.
- *Protein foods*. Allow yourself two portions of lean meat, fish or poultry (without the skin) or low fat dairy foods per day.
- *Fruit and vegetables*. Choose at least three helpings of each every day. Make sure they are fresh and clean.
- *Drink plenty of clean (filtered or bottled) water*. Supplement with herbal teas or slim-line drinks.
- *Use olive oil, sunflower oil or peanut oil for cooking*. Don't feel you have to cut out these fats – they are very good for you. But watch the calories!

Tips for losing weight

Using relaxation and visual imagery

One of the biggest problems in losing weight is motivation. It is all very well a doctor saying it should be done for the 'good of your health' or to keep at bay a complication in the future, but is this enough?

Researchers in New Zealand, recognizing the problems facing overweight diabetics, launched a study to find out if they could help diabetics modify their eating habits and lose weight. In the study, 27 Type II diabetics were asked to:

- record their daily food intake
- take up low impact and mild exercise sessions
- start relaxation classes
- identify stimuli to eating
- use visual imagery exercises to help control over-eating.

Over 11 weeks the group lost an average of 9.7 pounds (4.4 kilograms) each, and blood sugar levels and cholesterol levels both fell.

Using acupuncture
Probably the hardest part of dieting for anyone who is very overweight is overcoming hunger pangs. A person who over-eats has a stretched stomach and it does not take kindly to being asked to remain empty while it slowly contracts to the proper size.

Over-eating, especially comfort eating, is an ingrained habit as hard to break as any other. Hunger pangs are probably the main reason why many quite determined people have abandoned a reasonable, not to say essential, weight-loss programme.

But there is an easy answer: acupuncture, properly applied, removes hunger pangs by stimulating the release of the so-called 'pleasure hormones', *endorphins* and *encephalins*, which food also stimulates.

So, because acupuncture does the work of food, your stomach does not miss it and the pangs do not appear. Moreover, specialists in the technique claim that the effects last after the course of the acupuncture is over.

Social eating guide
Food and drinks which contain a lot of sugar (which should be avoided in any healthy diet, anyway) can pose

problems by causing blood sugar levels to spiral too quickly.

But, contrary to popular myth, you do not need to avoid sugar or sucrose completely. Research has shown that sucrose, when eaten on its own, produces a *glycaemic response* similar to bread, rice and potatoes.

The glycaemic response is the way blood glucose levels rise in response to different foods. The Glycaemic Index (see *figure 5*) gives a figure for each type of food. It has been devised by comparing the blood glucose rise caused by the foods against the response caused by an equivalent amount of glucose. Diabetics should not control their diet using the Glycaemic Index – it is only an indication of how food affects the body.

Christmas, birthdays and other feast days need not become too hard to manage if diabetes is well controlled. Insulin-dependent diabetics need to adjust their insulin requirements to cover special events, but do not need to miss out altogether. A small piece of cake or treat is best eaten at the end of a meal, rather than on its own, so that other food eaten will help to slow down the rate of absorption.

The diabetic's kitchen cupboard should contain:

- plenty of fresh fruit and vegetables
- low fat dairy products
- olive oil
- enough low fat protein such as chicken, turkey or beans to provide 10 to 20 (maximum) per cent of daily energy requirements.
- plenty of foods rich in fibre and starch such as oat bran cereals and crackers

What about diabetic foods?
Avoid at all costs. In 1992 the British Diabetic Association issued a report condemning 'diabetic foods' such as jams, chocolate and biscuits.

Grain, cereal products	%	Pulses	%
Buckwheat	51	Beans (tinned, baked)	40
Bread (white)	69	Beans (butter)	36
Bread (wholemeal)	72	Beans (haricot)	31
Millet	71	Beans (kidney)	29
Pastry	59	Beans (soya)	15
Rice (brown)	66	Beans (tinned, soya)	14
Rice (white)	72	Peas (blackeye)	33
Spaghetti (wholemeal)	42	Peas (chick)	36
Spaghetti (white)	50	Peanuts	13
Sweetcorn	59	Lentils	29

Breakfast cereals		Fruit	
All-bran	52	Apples	
Cornflakes	80	(golden delicious)	39
Muesli	66	Bananas	62
Porridge oats	49	Oranges	40
Shredded wheat	67	Orange juice	46
Weetabix	75	Raisins	64

Biscuits		Sugars	
Digestive	59	Fructose	20
Oatmeal	54	*Glucose*	*100*
Rich tea	55	Maltose	105
Ryvita	69	Sucrose	59
		Honey	87
Vegetables		Mars Bars	68
Broad beans	79	Lucozade	95
Frozen peas	51		

Root vegetables		Dairy products	
Beetroot	64	Ice cream	36
Carrots	92	Milk (skimmed)	32
Parsnips	97	Milk (whole)	34
Potato (instant)	80	Yoghurt	36
Potato (new)	70		
Swede	72		
Yam	51		

The above figures are based on a comparison against glucose as the standard 100%.

Fig. 5 The Glycaemic Index of common foods
From the *Optimum Nutrition Workbook* (see *Further Reading*)

They were introduced in the 1960s when diabetics were advised to cut down on carbohydrates and avoid sucrose – dietary advice which has now changed. In 1989 sales of diabetic foods were estimated to be worth £15 million ($22 million) in Britain but, in general, diabetic foods contain more fat and only slightly less energy than other comparable foods – and they cost up to four times as much!

The British Diabetic Association said: 'In terms of composition, diabetic foods remain an outmoded relic from an era of carbohydrate avoidance.'

Tips on drinking
Having diabetes does not mean giving up alcohol, although, if you are taking insulin, alcohol can make you more prone to having a hypo.

The advice is to have something to eat with your drink, preferably high-fibre foods, such as a wholemeal sandwich, which are more slowly digested and cause a more controlled rise in your blood sugar, and remember the following:

- Alcohol-free drinks tend to have a high sugar content: treat them like a sugared drink.
- Low-sugar beers tend to have a higher alcohol content.

Too much alcohol is not good for anyone's health. In diabetes as in anything, moderation is the key.

Alcohol consumption guide

Women   2 units a day/14 units a week maximum
Men   3 units a day/21 units a week maximum

(1 unit = 1 ordinary glass of wine/1 measure of spirit/1 half pint of beer)

Try to have two or three alcohol-free days each week.

Exercise

The British Diabetes Research Laboratory in Oxford, UK, is currently looking at whether exercise can alter and improve blood sugar levels among people with IGT and whether it lessens the likehood that they will go on to develop diabetes.

The theory is that taking action to lower blood sugar levels in the 'pre-diabetic' phase may well delay the onset of the disease and significantly reduce the risks of the disease's later complications.

Exercise can help lower blood sugar levels and encourage insulin to work more efficiently in the body and will also:

- give you more energy
- improve your circulation
- strengthen your muscles
- improve your breathing
- delay the effects of ageing
- improve cholesterol levels by lowering the 'bad' sort and raising the 'good'
- improve your personal 'feel good' factor
- delay or prevent heart disease

Exercise is a key to improved health because diabetes is all about the body's metabolism – how it captures and uses energy. Exercising for 20 to 30 minutes three times a week can trigger an increase in the number of insulin receptors, mainly on muscle cells, which then do a better job at attracting insulin during and after exercise. Clinical trials have shown that some forms of exercise such as yoga (see *Chapter 8*) have a very positive influence on diabetes, and can help to cause long-term reductions in blood glucose levels.

Insulin resistance is normally associated with Type II diabetes, but insulin-dependent diabetics can also become resistant, and this happens when insulin requirements rise to deal with everyday food intake.

The benefits of exercise for Type II diabetics

- Blood sugar is closer to normal, allowing you to be more flexible about food choices.
- You may be able to reduce or cut out oral medication to lower blood glucose.
- The pancreas does not need to produce as much insulin, which might delay the need for injected insulin.
- You should lose weight.

The benefits for Type I diabetics

- Blood sugar peaks can be minimized, particularly after meals.
- Insulin dosages can be reduced (only after careful monitoring).

Important guidelines for Type I diabetics

When non-diabetics exercise, insulin release from the pancreas shuts down but diabetics injecting insulin can't shut off the supply.

The vital thing about exercising is to avoid low blood sugar levels. Too much insulin circulating in the bloodstream can result in a hypo.

The simple solution is to eat some extra carbohydrate *or* reduce the dose of the injection before exercising.

Exercise has an individual effect on every person and depends on the type of exercise, duration, and your own age and weight.

As a guideline, for gentle exercise such as light gardening you will need an extra 10 milligrams of carbohydrate before you start and an extra 10-15 milligrams when you finish. This could be:

- a small apple or peach
- 7 dried apricot halves

- ¼ pint (1 cup) of a soft drink
- a digestive biscuit
- a small bag of crisps

For *strenuous exercise* such as an hour's tennis you may need 30-40 milligrams before you start and approximately 15 milligrams more every half hour or so. For example, a bowl of cereal, a healthy snack bar, or a low-fat wholemeal bread sandwich should do.

At the end you will need a smaller snack as the blood sugar level might continue to drop for some time after the exercise has been completed.

Andrew's story

'I was diagnosed as an insulin-dependent diabetic on Christmas Eve 1969. I was 14 years old, and it changed the course of my life. I suddenly had to cope with having injections. I was also told to be careful about what I ate and not to take part in competitive sports.

'As I grew up I realized I *could* take part in sports – and that it would be good for me. In the 1980s I joined the local athletics club. Today I run a marathon once a year, run in races most weeks during the season, climb mountains, compete in triathlon events, cycle, enjoy offshore swimming and work out in my own home gym.

'I am not sure whether I would have taken up sport if I had not become a diabetic. I am very competitive within myself, but it may also have had something to do with the fact that I was told I could not do sport when I was a boy.'

Andrew is now 40 and a member of the International Diabetics Athletes Association, racing internationally at every opportunity.

Weaving sport into his life on a daily basis, he believes, helps him control his diabetes. He keeps his weight stable, and the exercise encourages improved insulin control – his body accepts and uses the insulin better. He needs to monitor his blood glucose levels carefully and work out how and when he should exercise.

At work
Andrew is a chartered architect but finds time to exercise every day for an hour, doing a minimum of 30 minutes aerobics workout. A typical day is:

7am Blood test (average 12 mmol/l – see box *page 59* for an explanation of these measurements) followed by injection of 10 units of Actrapid, a short-acting insulin injected by pen device.
7.30am Breakfast of high fibre toast.
10am A snack, one banana.
12.30pm Finger prick blood test to check blood glucose level (average 8mmol/l) followed by next injection of 10 units of insulin.
1pm Lunch, high fibre sandwich, followed by fruit and yoghurt.
3.30pm Snack time, cereal bar.
6.30pm Finger prick blood test followed by 12 units of insulin in preparation for main meal of the day.
7pm Main meal of pasta and vegetables, followed by yoghurt and fruit.
10.30pm Last check of blood levels before bed and final injection of the day – this time 10 units of a longer-lasting insulin for night time cover followed by a snack of cereal and milk.

At play

On the day of a marathon run Andrew has to plan his daily routine differently to take into account his higher energy requirements. If the marathon is to begin at 9am the day will be as follows:

7am Check blood glucose levels with finger prick test. Inject 4 units of fast-acting insulin.

7.10am Breakfast on four thick slices of white toast with honey and a drink of water.

9am Marathon begins. After 5 to 8 miles (8 to 13 kilometres) Andrew will make sure he has a sugary drink. After 14–18 miles (22–30 kilometres), more of the same drink. After 22–26 miles (35–42 kilometres), a further sweet drink to boost glucose levels. The insulin plus exercise work to lower blood glucose levels, and the risk is they will drop too low and he will suffer a hypo. At 23 miles (37 kilometres), ¾ ounce (20 grams) of chocolate supplemented by water every 5 miles (8 kilometres) to prevent dehydration.

2pm Cross the finishing line and pig out on biscuits.

3pm Indulge in a large bowl of pasta.

5pm Enjoy a large bowl of cereal (carbohydrate to prevent blood glucose levels falling too low through insulin injection and through use of energy in the run).

10.30pm Andrew would expect his blood glucose levels to be around 14 mmol/l and the following morning 16 mmol/l. He aims to keep his glucose levels high to avoid a 'mega hypo', a result of low blood sugar levels. This is the danger for diabetics taking part in an exhausting sport, and the risk of a hypo remains for about three days afterwards.

In summary

- Aerobic exercise improves insulin sensitivity: choose from walking, swimming, cycling, jogging, rowing or aerobics.
- The goal is 20 to 45 minutes of continuous activity plus a 5 to 10 minute warm-up and cool-down period.
- Be prepared to monitor blood sugar levels frequently during the first months of a new exercise programme.

Stress management

Dr Clare Bradley, reader in healing psychology at the University of London, has studied stress and diabetes for many years, and says that stress can both trigger diabetes and disrupt control of the disease. It is important that diabetics learn to recognize their own stressors, and then take appropriate action.

You can do this by:

- making up a chart of things that bother or concern you
- checking blood levels before and after a potentially stressful situation (an interview, a visit to the dentist)
- keeping a chart to jot down your reactions and see if a pattern develops
- taking evasive action by making an effort to relax using a gentle therapy *before* the stressful situation.

If you are a Type I diabetic and you note your blood glucose levels *fall* because of stress, you can prepare in advance by eating some extra carbohydrate. Stress and stress management techniques are explored in more detail in *Chapter 8*.

Thoughts, feelings and moods can influence your stress levels. If you sense a negative mood coming on, slip a rubber band over your wrist. Each time a worrying thought crops up 'ping' the rubber band to try and stop those thoughts. Attempt to replace the thought with a positive or good thought or try a favourite poem or positive mental image.

This technique can help you to train yourself to stop the negative thoughts which can be triggers to feelings of stress.

What to do next

Though self-help techniques such as diet and exercise can help considerably in the management of diabetes, they are not frontline treatments. Normally the sort of safe, gentle and effective treatments you want will be offered by a natural therapist rather than a doctor. Nevertheless when diabetes is diagnosed, the first port of call will not normally be a natural therapist and it is more likely you will be instructed in treating your diabetes by your family doctor. The following chapter explains what he or she is likely to say and do and also what is generally on offer for diabetes conventionally.

CHAPTER 5

Conventional treatments and procedures

What your doctor is likely to say and do

When you turn up at the family doctor's centre with all the symptoms of diabetes you should be taken very seriously from the start.

You might go to the doctor with your own suspicions. You might have been drinking more and more and getting thirsty at night, and frequently visiting the bathroom to pass water.

Or you could be 'picked up' through routine Well Man or Well Woman clinic tests. A urine test will reveal high levels of glucose in the system, but this is only a warning bell. Urine tests cannot be used to diagnose diabetes, only to tip off the doctor that further investigation would be a good idea.

If symptoms are present the doctor will want to confirm his or her diagnosis of diabetes with a blood test. This may be carried out in hospital, at a specialist diabetes clinic or at the doctor's own practice.

If there is any doubt that your condition is caused by diabetes your doctor will want to run two separate tests to confirm the suspicions, and to find out whether it really is diabetes, or is impaired glucose tolerance – which at present requires no conventional treatment apart from regular monitoring.

In addition to the blood test, a further urine test will routinely be carried out to look for the presence of *ketones*. This, in conjunction with a blood test, will diagnose Type I diabetes. As explained earlier, ketones are a byproduct of burning fat for energy and a sign that no insulin is being produced. Instead the body has turned to the fat cells for vital fuel to keep going.

Different types of test

A *random blood test* might be taken at your first visit to the surgery. This will give a good idea as to the levels of glucose flowing in the blood, but might not be completely accurate if, for example, you have just eaten a meal.

A *fasting blood test* is carried out after 12 hours of fasting. Early in the morning is the usual time for such a test.

The *Glucose Tolerance Test* (GTT) might be offered to people with no symptoms of diabetes or if you are considered to be a 'borderline diabetic'. It involves drinking 2½ ounces (75 grams) of pure glucose dissolved in water and having blood tests on the hour or half hour for the following two hours. This test diagnoses:

- diabetes
- impaired glucose tolerance
- normal insulin production, coping as expected with the influx of glucose.

In healthy individuals glucose concentrations rise to about twice the normal level in the first hour and return to normal within two hours. In diabetics the blood glucose rises to a much higher level, the return to normal is delayed and a large amount of glucose is excreted in the urine.

Another test you may hear about is called a *glycosylated haemoglobin test* and gives doctors a longer-term view

of your condition. The test can tell from your haemoglobin (the chemical which makes your blood cells red)
how well the glucose/insulin balance has been working
in previous weeks and may be performed two or three
times a year. A new machine called the 'Glycomat' produced by Drew Scientific received American approval in
1994 and this makes the test far easier and cheaper to
organize, as well as providing the scope for more frequent tests.

How blood tests show diabetes

Blood tests show what level of glucose there is in the blood.
In most countries except America this is now measured in
'millimoles per litre', written 'mmol/l'. (In America the old
measure 'milligrams per decilitre' or 'mg/dl' is still used.) For
example, a normal blood glucose level is anything below 7.8
mmol/l, whether you have fasted or just eaten. The World
Health Organization guidelines say that diabetes is established when the glucose levels in the blood are over 11
mmol/l during a glucose tolerance test. In some out-of-con-
trol diabetes the levels can soar as high as 30. *Figure 6*
shows what the different levels mean.

If you are diagnosed with diabetes you are entitled to
see a specialist trained in diabetes care. You might find
that 'shared care' with your family doctor and specialist
is the best way forward.

Once a diagnosis is confirmed, a specialist will want
to make a full physical examination to determine:

- if any other disease has caused the onset of diabetes
  (for example, a disease of the pancreas)
- if any of the diabetic complications already mentioned
  in this book have set in, and if so whether to start a
  treatment plan

TARGETS FOR DIABETICS

		Good	Acceptable	Poor	Very poor
Blood fats					
Total cholesterol (HDL/LDL)	mmol/l	under 5.2	5.2 – 6.4	6.5 – 7.8	over 7.8
	mg/dl (US)	under 150	150 – 200	200 – 240	over 240
Triglycerides	mmol/l	under 1.7	1.7 – 2.2	2.3 – 4.4	over 4.4
	md/dl (US)	under 100	100 – 120	200 – 250	over 250
Blood pressure					
Systolic pressure	mmHg	under 140	140 – 159	160 – 180	over 180
Diastolic pressure	mmHg	under 90	91 – 94	95 – 100	over 100

Please note The above figures are for guidance only. Total cholesterol is not as significant a reading as those for high density lipoprotein (HDL) cholesterol and low density lipoprotein (LDL) cholesterol separately. The higher the HDL and the lower the LDL the better. Blood pressure also varies quite normally depending on age, sex, time of the day and emotions and activities during the day. An average of several readings should always be taken over a period of time for an accurate indication.

Fig. 6 Targets for diabetics

If you are taking any natural remedies, tell your doctor at this stage as a courtesy. Some traditional remedies such as *karela*, an Asian fruit (see *Chapter 9*), do lower blood glucose levels and this will have an impact on your test results.

The medical examination will find out whether you are dehydrated, will check your heart and circulation through pulse and blood pressure checks, check your lungs and breathing, abdomen, nervous system and senses. The doctor may want to look at your feet and ask about joints and ligaments. You may also be offered a blood cholesterol test as blood fats can be raised in untreated diabetes.

Myths about diabetes

● Diabetes is *not* caused by eating too much sugar.
● Diabetes is *not* life-threatening: with proper management you can lead a normal, long life.
● Diabetes does *not* prevent you having children: you can go on to have a family.
● Diabetes does *not* mean you can no longer enjoy yourself: you don't have to stop enjoying your life or your food.
● Diabetes does *not* mean you are handicapped: you can go on holiday, work and carry on as normal.

Coping with the diagnosis

Being diagnosed as a diabetic can lead to all sorts of feelings of guilt, sorrow, anger, despair, and shock. But often this is more out of ignorance of the condition than anything. Because diabetes is such a complex and complicated disease there is a great deal of ignorance about it amongst people generally.

On the other hand, don't expect to come to terms with diabetes overnight. It will take time. If you are a parent, feelings of guilt and fears for the future are all normal, natural reactions. These will slowly disperse as you find out more about the condition, and what you can do to help yourself and your family.

Treatment

If you are diagnosed as a Type I diabetic you will immediately be prescribed the only treatment available: insulin.

Insulin is a protein and so cannot be given in tablet form. It would be digested by the stomach and made inactive.

The only way to give insulin is by injection. As a parent you will be taught how to give your child injections (see *Chapter 3*). Very fine needles are now available for this as well as special pen injectors and these make the whole process simple, quick and virtually pain free.

The dose of insulin is tailor-made to each individual, taking into account lifestyle, height, weight and age.

In the beginning it might be very much trial and error and you will probably be asked to carry out a number of blood glucose tests at home to see whether enough insulin is being injected to keep glucose levels stable.

The aim is to restore insulin levels to as near normal as possible, so instead of having high blood sugar levels of 10 mmol/l and above, you would expect regularly to see something below 7 mmol/l.

The basic equation is a balancing act, juggling the insulin intake with food and exercise (see *figure 7*). As a rule of thumb food makes the glucose level rise, exercise and insulin make it fall.

Your doctor will explain to you about your individual dose of insulin. If you radically change your lifestyle by taking up more exercise and eating different foods talk to the doctor.

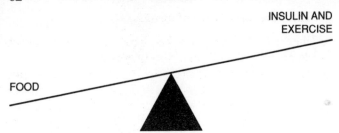

Fig. 7 Balancing food with insulin and exercise

The most common 'regimes' or treatment programmes are:

- a single dose of long-acting insulin (only really used with elderly patients)
- a twice-daily injection, a combination of short- and medium-acting insulin. This provides day and night cover and means eating at set, regular times.
- a four times a day injection with short-acting insulin before meals and a medium or long-lasting insulin at bed time. This system provides more flexibility in eating times.

Types of insulin

Insulin treatments have made tremendous strides in the past two decades. There are now 38 different types of insulin currently available in the UK alone. The majority of diabetics use 'human' insulin, which is genetically engineered in a laboratory and not derived from human tissue. It is easier to produce and is 'purer' than insulin from animal sources. However, some 25 per cent of diabetics use animal insulin, derived from pigs or cows which have been slaughtered for human consumption.

As a resul diabetics are being given far more freedom from the restrictions of regular meals, timed to the hour, than ever before.

There are three types of insulin:

- *long-lasting,* which gives 'background' cover, for example overnight, and has a cloudy appearance
- *short-acting,* which is clear, and can be injected 20 minutes before a meal to 'cover' the food that will be eaten
- *mixed,* also of cloudy appearance and containing both
- in addition, there is ongoing development and research of a new fast-acting insulin which can be taken 5 minutes before eating.

Insulin is given by:

- traditional *syringe*
- insulin *pens* which are pre-loaded with cartridges of insulin and have very fine needles incorporated into the gadget (see *figure 8*)
- *pumps* which inject insulin automatically

Other ways of taking insulin

For people with needle phobias preliminary studies in America show some success with inhaling insulin through the nose or mouth. The amounts needed to work are higher than those given by injection but there is every indication this method could be more widely available in the near future.

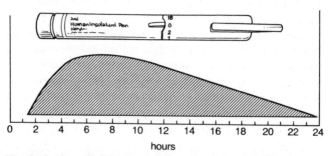

Fig. 8 An insulin injector 'pen' and graph showing a time-action profile

Figure 9 gives a list of the most common insulin preparations and their action.

	Synonyms	**Appearance**	**Pattern of use**
Short-acting	Soluble	Clear	With meals
Medium-acting	Isophane Semilente Lente	Cloudy	Once/twice daily
Long-acting	Ultralente Protamine	Cloudy	Once/twice daily
Pre-mixed	Biphasic	Cloudy	Twice daily

Fig. 9 Common insulin preparations

Treatment for Type II diabetics

If your blood glucose levels are high, and you have been diagnosed as a Type II diabetic, you may be given tablets to lower blood glucose levels. They are called *hypoglycaemic drugs* – or drugs to stimulate insulin production. There are three different groups :

Sulphonylureas

These work by stimulating insulin release from the pancreas. They might encourage weight gain and are usually prescribed to diabetics who have been unable to control their diabetes by diet alone. Common types are glibenclamide, gliclazide, glipizide, tolbutamide and chlorpropamide. The drawback is the risk of suffering hypos when blood sugar levels drop too low. As with Type I diabetics, attention has to be paid to the balance of food input against energy expenditure.

Biguanides

This is a class of drug that helps lower blood glucose levels and is usually offered to overweight diabetics who have not been able to achieve 'diabetic control' by diet alone. There can be side-effects of nausea and diarrhoea, and it is recommended they are taken with food.

Alpha glucosidase inhibitors

A new type of drug is prescribed when diet alone is not enough to control high blood sugar levels. These drugs work by slowing down the digestion and the absorption of carbohydrates into the bloodstream.

Insulin will be prescribed for Type II diabetics if:

- symptoms continue – especially lack of energy
- there is continuing weight loss
- there are persistent ketone levels found in the urine

Diet and exercise for Type II diabetics

As already explained in *Chapter 4*, a large proportion of Type II diabetics will be able to control their diabetes by diet alone. Though you can do this for yourself, most areas now have specialist diabetic nurses on call to answer immediate worries and problems. Once diagnosed, you will be asked for regular medical checkups and blood tests to monitor the progress of the disease.

Surgery

Experimental techniques for treating diabetes surgically are now under development in both Britain and America, though they are not regarded as frontline treatment yet. They are:

- *Islet cell transplantation* (ICT)
- *Pancreas transplantation*

Islet cell transplantation

By 1995 a total of 150 diabetics worldwide had been treated with islet cell transplantation, a procedure that involves transplanting healthy insulin-producing cells from the pancreas directly into the liver. It is a 20-minute process, performed under a local anaesthetic. Blood in the liver encourages cells to settle and start producing insulin in the normal way, as they would in the pancreas.

The first operation was carried out in America in 1989 and a total of six had been performed in Britain by 1995. But the results are still far from satisfactory. The longest any patient has been able to remain off insulin treatment after an islet cell transplant is three years.

The aim is to perfect the technique, and offer this as a treatment for newly diagnosed diabetics to prevent the disease and its complications from developing.

Pancreas transplantation

Pancreas transplantation is the most radical form of treatment for diabetes. There has been some success with this operation but it carries risks and is a difficult procedure.

As a result, it is presently only offered to diabetics who are suffering serious kidney complications and need a kidney transplant. The pancreas transplant is carried out at the same time.

Though there have been success stories, it is seen very much as a 'last resort' treatment. Patients might be able to give up insulin but they have to continue taking strong anti-rejection drugs instead.

Problems with conventional treatment

- It is difficult to keep to the 'tight control' which is currently recommended.
- As many as 36 per cent of people lose their sensitivity or warning signs to hypoglycaemia if they change from animal to human insulin.

● This loss of sensitivity means that even tighter controls
  – that is, more glucose testing – have to be carried out
  more frequently. This can create a vicious circle of testing and feelings of failure or stress if you are unable to
  keep to recommended glucose levels.

Summary

For the newly diagnosed diabetic, the message from conventional practitioners will be to test regularly to check
on how blood glucose levels are faring. You will soon
see a pattern emerging so you can judge the level
required to keep you in control of the situation.

Keeping blood glucose levels in harmony cuts the
risks of later complications by more than half, so there is
good reason to do this.

In the next few chapters we look at ways to complement conventional treatment. That is, how other remedies might be used in tandem with the medicines and
advice given by your doctor or diabetes specialist, and
so give you the best chance of managing your diabetes
safely, gently and effectively.

CHAPTER SIX

The natural therapies and diabetes

Introducing the 'gentle alternatives'

For many people with Type II diabetes, a change in diet and lifestyle may be all that is needed to banish their symptoms and stabilize their disease – though most diabetics will continue to need regular monitoring.

But for both Type I and Type II diabetics there will be times when extra help is needed to keep blood glucose levels stable: at times of stress, for example, or to alleviate the very unpleasant, painful and difficult problems caused by complications of the disease.

So where to turn? By now you will probably be all too familiar with conventional medicine's strategy for coping with diabetes. Doctors tend to follow the progression from diet and exercise to hypoglycaemic drugs to insulin, for Type II diabetes.

By now you may be ready to try something different, something that will complement your conventional treatment and may even help it to work more efficiently.

If this is you, then you are in good company. Each year in the Western world thousands of people turn to natural therapies for virtually every health complaint under the sun – even diabetes, for which there is no cure.

The choice of natural therapy and therapist is in fact growing so fast that there is almost too much choice, and for some this alone can prove daunting. Where do you start? And how safe is it to follow alternative treatments with a disease like diabetes?

The first thing to realize is that if you want the fresh approach of a natural therapy but the security provided by a conventional doctor, that is by no means impossible these days.

More and more doctors are becoming converted to particular types of natural therapies and are incorporating them into their conventional practice. Dr Peter Fisher, a consultant at the Royal London Homoeopathic Hospital who completed a study of complementary medicine throughout Europe in 1994, says that in the last 20 years what he terms the 'Big Five' – acupuncture, herbalism, homoeopathy, osteopathy and chiropractic – have become so common they are virtually orthodox.

This is even more the case in America and in continental Europe. In France more than 80 per cent of herbal medicines are prescribed by doctors while in Belgium 84 per cent of homoeopathy and 74 per cent of acupuncture are carried out by family doctors.

The next few chapters will, hopefully, provide an insight into what is available, and from whom, and what it can do for diabetes and its complications.

What is natural therapy?

Natural therapy is based on the belief that the body has a natural, built-in ability to heal itself and that the fundamental aim of any treatment is to bolster and enhance this ability.

A natural therapist looks at illness and disease with a different perspective from a conventional medical practitioner. The emphasis is on applying a treatment to boost the body's defences and build up resistance so that your body does the healing itself in its own way and in its own time.

The natural therapist will want to look at your lifestyle, your general health, and your state of mind. To him or her, the whole person rather than the physical body is important. That means natural therapists want to restore harmony in the mind and emotions as well the body.

The reason for this is that natural therapists believe that the human body is not simply a physical machine to be mended like a car, but a complex blend of body, mind and emotions, or soul if you prefer – any one or all of which can cause or contribute to health problems.

Apart from this all-important difference there are a number of other important beliefs and principles that underlie natural therapies and distinguish them from most conventional medical approaches. They can be summarized as follows:

- True healing can only take place when the root cause of the problem is identified.
- Good health is a state of physical, mental and emotional, or spiritual, balance. This principle of balance as central to the idea of health in natural medicine finds expression in Chinese medicine, for example, as the principle of *yin* and *yang*.
- There is a natural healing force in the universe that anyone can make use of, but it is the natural therapist's role in particular to activate this force or help patients activate it for themselves. The Chinese call this force *qi* or *chi*, the Japanese *ki*, and the Indians *prana*.
- People heal more quickly if they take responsibility for their own health and play an active role in the therapeutic process – unlike the traditionally 'passive' role taken by patients in conventional medicine.
- Environmental and social factors have an extremely powerful influence on people's health and can be as important as their physical or psychological makeup.

● Each person is an individual and therefore different people may need different treatments.

You may think quite a lot of this sounds extremely sensible – so why don't more conventional doctors subscribe to these principles? The answer is they do, but without necessarily subscribing to some of the Oriental philosophy behind it.

There are many good conventional doctors who do build up much the same sort of healing relationship with their patients as natural therapists do. But rather than talk about *chi* they would simply say that there is a strong basic tendency for orderliness in the universe and our own natural self-healing abilities are one example of it.

The reason most doctors still do not accept the majority of natural therapies is because they are based on ideas – like *chi* – that do not fit into conventional scientific understanding.

Reflexology, for example, involves massaging the feet in order to stimulate healing in specific organs elsewhere in the body. Thousands of satisfied customers testify that it helps them, but a doctor trained in anatomy finds it very hard to believe.

The fact that a therapy appears to be able to defy the laws of science as they are presently understood, and still work, is something many conventionally trained doctors and scientists are simply unable to accept.

The advantages of the natural therapies

Arguably the greatest of the advantages of natural medicine over conventional medicine is the close relationship established between therapist and patient. The simple act of consultation with a good practitioner can be healing in itself. Some conventional doctors manage this with their patients but many more don't. Yet this relationship is often the key to discovering the underlying problems that are at the root of ill-health.

Another advantage is that alternative therapies, unlike drugs and most conventional medical techniques, are generally non-invasive and free of side-effects. This becomes an important consideration, especially when dealing with a disease like diabetes which is incurable but, for the most part, controllable.

Conventional medical drugs effectively aim to *control* diabetes. Natural remedies, by contrast, try to *channel* the disease. That is, they try to enhance the body's natural powers of recovery to such a degree that some of these medicines might either no longer be required, or have their dosage reduced (*but be careful – do not do this without the agreement and co-operation of your doctor*).

Most natural therapies are very pleasant, especially those involving touch and massage. As we have already learned, relaxation is a wonderful way to help lower blood glucose levels.

Unlike many conventional treatments, natural therapies have side-effects that are almost entirely positive. Many people with no specific health problems book regular sessions of 'touch' therapies simply for the sheer feeling of well-being these therapies bring.

Many people who try a natural therapy for a specific physical problem find as a result that they are more relaxed and positive about life in general and that their self-image is much improved.

How natural therapies treat diabetes

Although all natural therapies share the fundamental holistic principles outlined above, in practice they can be divided into two fairly distinct categories: psychological therapies and physical therapies.

Psychological therapies aim to treat your mental and emotional condition while physical therapies concentrate on your physical state. For instance, hypnotherapy and meditation are clearly aimed at your psychological state, while manipulative therapies such as massage are hands-on physical treatments for your body.

Of course, there are huge areas of overlap. Improving your mental state will help improve your overall health as well, either through the direct effects of relaxation or because you become more positive and change aspects of your lifestyle and attitudes that may be adversely affecting your health.

By the same token, improving your physical health will have a similarly positive effect on your mental state and emotions for, as we have already seen, the two are inseparable.

Then there are therapies which set out to treat mind and body at the same time. Techniques such as yoga are excellent exercise for your whole body but they also have a strong psychological effect.

The dual approach makes natural therapies helpful and useful adjuncts to managing diabetes. For example, psychological therapy such as hypnosis or biofeedback can help sufferers come to terms with their disease and perhaps view it in a more positive way. Type I diabetes is for life, so this form of natural therapy can be used to help diabetics face up to the future positively.

It may, in some cases, even help to reduce symptoms and deal with some of the suffering caused by complications affecting the nerves, eyes, kidneys and heart.

Meanwhile, a physical approach, using new 'functional foods' or acupuncture, can alleviate symptoms and help to create physiological changes, such as reductions in blood glucose levels and altering lipid levels in the blood. This, in turn, will help you gain more control over diabetes rather than allowing diabetes to control you.

Natural therapies helpful for diabetes

Psychological therapies	*Physical therapies*
Autogenics	Aromatherapy
Biofeedback	Functional foods
Counselling	Herbal medicine
Creative visualization	Homoeopathy
Deep relaxation	Hydrotherapy
Hypnotherapy	Massage
Meditation	Naturopathic medicine
	Reflexology
	Traditional Oriental medicines
	Yoga

Summary

Natural therapies can help to:

- treat your psychological condition to counter stress
- treat your overall physical condition and increase your level of well-being

In the management of diabetes they do this by:

- counteracting, reducing and eliminating psychological strain through relaxation
- helping to identify behaviour and habits that put you at risk of unnecessary swings in blood glucose
- stimulate the body's natural regenerative processes
- tone up tissues and organs
- improve circulation (good for those suffering disorders of the nervous system)
- help lower levels of fat and glucose in the bloodstream

In the next few chapters we shall look at how the therapies listed above can help. (For how to find and choose a natural therapist, see *Chapter 10*.)

CHAPTER 7

Treating your mind and emotions

Managing diabetes and stress

The more medical science looks into the way body and mind are linked, the more evidence there is that the mind does have a profound influence on almost every disease investigated. It is only in relatively recent times that Western cultures have considered the treatment of body, mind and spirit in isolation from each other.

Having a calm interior (the mind) can influence the exterior (the body). Inner turmoil may affect diabetes because of the impact that stress hormones can have on blood glucose levels, causing high or low swings, and on skin blood flow, which can affect insulin absorption rates.

There is some evidence in Type I diabetes, for example, that long-term stress or major life stressors can actually speed up the antibody attack on the insulin-producing cells, triggering an earlier onset of the disease.

Defining stress

Stress is very individual. We all react differently to sets of circumstances, and having diabetes can add to the psychological strain of dealing with common experiences such as marriage, birth and bereavement.

In general, stress causes our body to behave as if it were under attack. We can react positively to this, by becoming energized and motivated, or we can react negatively by failing to adapt to external or internal pressures.

Stress comes in all shapes, forms and sizes. It might be physical such as injury, illness or the diagnosis of diabetes, or it might be psychological like marriage problems, divorce, bereavement or redundancy.

Then there are everyday stresses. These might be as simple as the washing-machine breaking down, the car not starting or missing a bus.

How we react is also very individual. We all have our threshold, the limit to the amount of stress our minds and bodies can take. An overload of stresses – more than we can handle – can cause feelings of tension and anxiety to mount.

We may then find ourselves in the black foothills of anxiety, succumbing to panic, unable to concentrate, unable to function properly or effectively. Out of control feelings of worry, frustration, hostility, anger and resentment develop.

Being 'stressed' probably means you are feeling 'uptight', tense, unnaturally wound up, and feeling incapable of letting go, relaxing, letting life flow along as it should. It is a combination of both strain and tension.

When we are under stress the body prepares to take action. This is called our 'fight or flight' response and dates back to the days of our prehistoric ancestors.

Levels of many hormones shoot up, and the effect is to make a lot of stored energy – glucose and fat – available to all cells to fuel the 'flight'.

For diabetics this fight or flight response might not work quite so well. Insulin may not work so efficiently in times of stress, and glucose levels can rise.

This is likely to be the case for Type II diabetics.

Laboratory tests among Type I diabetics have shown a more mixed response to stress. In the majority of cases blood glucose levels rise, but in some they stay the same – and in a smaller group levels actually fall.

In order to take action to combat stress – through relaxation or stress management programmes – it is important to know how you react to a stressful situation. One way is to keep a chart recording stressful situations and your reaction to them by comparing the rise or fall in blood glucose levels.

The effects of stress

In 1985 researchers in Australia followed up 1,526 people who survived the devastating bush fires of South Australia in 1983. The incidence of a number of disorders – including diabetes – 'significantly increased' 12 months after the fires.

In another study the same year British researchers investigated the background of 13 insulin-dependent diabetics and found 77 per cent had experienced one or more major life stresses in the three years before they were diagnosed.

The stress of having diabetes

A diagnosis of diabetes is a major source of stress as it means making major life changes. It is a disease which demands constant attention, and constant control.

Dr Richard Shillitoe, in his book *Counselling People with Diabetes*, describes developing the disease as a bit like entering into an arranged marriage from which there can be no divorce.

There might be many moments of harmony and amicable co-existence but also periods of disharmony and uncertainty.

If diabetes is diagnosed in middle age it will take a huge effort of will and motivation to change and adopt a new lifestyle. There will be considerable outside pressure to make those changes 'for your own good'.

For insulin-dependent diabetics the transition from 'normal' life to a highly organized, controlled and regimented lifestyle involving daily monitoring, set eating patterns, and regular injections can be extremely stressful.

Having diabetes might well affect your job (you cannot be an airline pilot, for example, if you are a diabetic); it certainly means being 'labelled' for life.

If you are insulin-dependent the conventional advice is to wear some form of identity bracelet, in case of diabetic coma or hypo. You will need to carry around a constant reminder of your condition if you are Type I diabetic: your daily equipment necessary for survival in the form of a syringe or an insulin injector pen.

It is not surprising, therefore, that diabetics or their parents can at times experience great feelings of frustration and anger, and ask the question, 'Why me?' or 'Why my child? Where did I go wrong?'

Internal stress and turmoil may contribute to a worsening of your condition, and diabetics can find themselves at certain times of their lives locked into a pattern of bad diabetes control and emotional suffering.

So we can see there is plenty of scope in the treatment of diabetes for gentle therapies which can soothe the mind, and by doing so enhance the control and management of the disease.

Amongst the therapies which have been found to be useful are:

- autogenic training
- biofeedback
- counselling
- hydrotherapy
- hypnotherapy
- meditation
- relaxation techniques
- visualization

Autogenic training

Autogenic training or 'autogenics' is a Westernized form of meditation that also includes the techniques of auto-suggestion. It is a *psycho-physiological* technique that involves both the mind and the body – and it is this that makes it different from other purely muscular relaxation methods.

The technique involves three basic parts: passive con-centration, mental repetition of a group of phrases asso-ciated with certain parts of the body and certain conditions (such as warmth and heaviness in the limbs, a calm and regular heartbeat, soothing abdominal warmth, and self-regulation of breathing), and, thirdly, the elimination of any arousing or disturbing stimuli.

The theory is that this is a form of self-hypnosis that can modify the body's natural self-regulatory (or *homoeo-static*) mechanisms, including the endocrine system. Learning autogenics takes 5 to 10 sessions of one hour each once a week – after which you are 'on your own' to use the system as required.

Autogenics involves a set of six specific mental exer-cises which are repeated and used to help cope with stressful situations.

Biofeedback

Biofeedback is a way of monitoring your own responses with special equipment.

For example, the machine might be linked up to mea-sure your heart rate. You might hear a series of beeps: the faster they are, the faster the beats. By making an effort to relax you learn to slow the heart beat, and feel the positive benefit. You also begin to understand your own feelings of tension.

Research has shown that using biofeedback techniques can improve blood flow and circulation particularly when it is coupled with relaxation tapes focusing on feelings of warmth and heaviness. This sort of technique might be helpful for diabetics with blood circulation problems or loss of feeling in the hands and feet.

Counselling

Counselling is a means of helping you to help yourself by exploring problems, clarifying them and encouraging you to make decisions about what to do next. This can be helpful if something is wrong or depressing you and you cannot seem to get to the bottom of it.

Counsellors need to have the skill to listen, convey warmth and interest, and ask open and direct questions. It is best to find someone familiar with diabetes, including the implications and complications, and you may find a diabetic counsellor on your healthcare team.

Counselling can empower you to understand more about your disease, the future and the best way to help yourself. Counsellors will encourage you to learn more about your diabetes, discuss sensitive subjects such as impotence, and furnish you with the skills for better self-management.

Sessions range from 15 to 45 minutes and you might find visits over a period of weeks are needed before you begin to experience real and lasting benefits.

Hydrotherapy

Hydrotherapy is again becoming fashionable after a period in the doldrums. Hydrotherapy means, literally, 'water therapy' and any form of therapy with water is hydrotherapy, including swimming.

Other forms are thalassotherapy – using sea water for a variety of ailments including circulatory disorders – and mineral spa baths. In many European countries, especially France and Germany, thalassotherapy centres are hugely popular for their restorative and healing powers and some employers recommend their staff to use annual leave for rejuvenating breaks at one of many centres found in both countries.

Another form of hydrotherapy popular in most Western countries is 'floating' in special 'flotation tanks' filled with just enough warm salt water to keep you afloat in a quiet, enclosed chamber. Floating is said to induce deep relaxation.

Yet another form of hydrotherapy is 'dolphin swimming' (see box).

Swimming with dolphins

Swimming with dolphins is fast becoming a fashionable as well as highly enjoyable relaxation technique. Places such as Eilat, in Israel, Bali, the Bahamas, Florida, Australia's Gold Coast, and parts of the coast around the British Isles now organize trips for visitors to swim amongst wild dolphins.

Marie Helene Roussel, a specialist in 're-birthing' techniques who organizes dolphin-swimming excursions to Israel from her base in London, says there is anecdotal evidence of many people, including diabetics, who have shown improvements in either physical or mental conditions after swimming with dolphins.

Hypnotherapy

Hypnotherapy, or hypnosis, is a well-researched and well-established therapy that has been shown to be able to help people with sometimes deeply entrenched fears and anxieties. Although there is no evidence that it will specifically help diabetes, studies have shown it can help soothe and calm the mind in times of emotional disturbance.

A hypnotherapist can help you deal with the emotional trauma and upset which lead to stress, and hypnosis offers the chance to enjoy deep relaxation.

A word of caution Because of its powerful nature it is important you see only a properly qualified and fully experienced practitioner and make quite sure you are happy with the person before you agree to treatment (see *Chapter 10*).

Meditation

Meditation is now a well tried and tested technique for dissolving feelings of tension and stress. It can induce deep rest, improve mental clarity and alertness, improve sleep patterns, and reduce stress, anxiety and depression.

To meditate at home, choose a quiet room and sit comfortably with hands resting loosely on your lap. The classic meditation pose is the 'lotus' position seen in Indian prints but you can actually sit in any way you find comfortable. It will be just as effective.

The aim is to clear your mind of all stimulating or troublesome thoughts. The simplest way to do this is to replace it with something else calming and still. For example, you could chant a word such as 'Om', 'God' or 'One'.

Repeat the word regularly and rhythmically. As you establish a rhythm, slow down the chanting (but speed it up if disturbing thoughts interfere with your concentration).

You can choose to focus on your breathing, or on an object such as a picture or a candle. By doing this, attention is focused inwards, bringing about an inner calm and awareness.

Though meditation can be learned and practised at home, it is not easy. There are a number of variations – *Transcendental Meditation* being one of the best known – but all take concentration and time to master properly and it is really best to get instruction from a trained teacher in the first place.

Psychotherapy

A form of counselling by another name, psychotherapy aims to understand and treat underlying mental and emotional problems without going to the extent of using trance techniques as in hypnotherapy, although some psychotherapists are also hypnotherapists.

There is a wide and almost bewildering variety of psychotherapeutic techniques available – from humanistic psychology to Freudian analysis – and it is impossible to say what is best for everyone in a book of this size.

The best advice, if you are interested in exploring this area, is to start by talking to a counsellor. They usually know most of the techniques and therapists around and can suggest a next step most likely to be helpful in your case.

Relaxation techniques

Some researchers make great claims of being able to lower blood glucose levels in stressed diabetics by the use of special relaxation techniques. Others say relaxation techniques have no effect at all.

One view suggests relaxation only helps Type II diabetics, yet others say they have had success with Type Is. At the end of the day it is a personal decision: 'you pays your money and takes your choice.' If it works for you and feels good, do it.

Relaxation aims to encourage a sense of deep inner

peace, promoting a sense of wellbeing and providing the tools needed to cope with repressed anger, hostility or resentment.

Relaxation may be as simple as a hot bath and a cup of camomile tea. Or it might be as 'high tech' as being connected to an electronic biofeedback machine to monitor tension in the body.

Even if it does not directly affect your diabetic condition, it might help relieve feelings of frustration and worry and simply help you to cope better with life.

At home you can boost relaxation by:

- exercising
- banishing negative thoughts
- replacing negative thoughts with positive ones
- setting aside 'me' time: time to walk, talk, listen to music and generally do things that *you* enjoy
- taking avoiding action – if a route to work means stressful traffic jams, change it
- listening to relaxation tapes

Relaxation tapes are used in progressive relaxation therapy and contain instructions on how to tense and then release or relax parts of the body. By the end of a 30-minute exercise you might find yourself drifting off to sleep. The tapes teach you to identify tension in your body, and by releasing the tension you learn how to relax.

The British Holistic Medical Association publishes audio-tapes for relaxation as part of its *Tapes for Health* series, as does the Yoga Biomedical Trust in London (see *Appendix A*).

Visualization

Visualization is a simple and sometimes highly effective technique that involves creating healing and health-promoting pictures in your own mind.

The technique has had some success among cancer patients taught to visualize the destruction of the cancer-forming cells in their bodies by healthy life-enhancing cells.

Other therapies

Other therapies that claim to treat psychological problems are:

- Homoeopathy (see *Chapter 8*)
- Flower remedies

Flower remedies
Flower remedies are made from the flowers of wild plants, bushes and trees but are not used to treat physical complaints directly, as are herbs. They are used more for treating states of mind or moods.

The theory is that as peace and harmony are restored so the body 'closes the circuit', allowing the 'life force' or *chi* to flow freely, promoting the body's natural healing.

The best known are the Bach flower remedies – named after the British homoeopath Dr Edward Bach who created the original range of 39 remedies in the 1920s and 30s – but there are now other varieties sold in America, Australia and Britain.

Examples of the Bach remedies are pine to treat guilt, olive for fatigue, walnut for helping in a move to new surroundings or circumstances, wild rose for apathy, and mustard for feeling sad and low for no apparent reason. A small size bottle will provide enough for about 45 treatments. It is concentrated, so you add a few drops to spring water which is sipped at intervals during the day.

Though there is no scientific evidence that they do what they claim, nor any explanation how they might work, many thousands of people around the world swear by their therapeutic effect.

CHAPTER 8

Treating physical symptoms

Physical therapies for diabetes

Physical therapies all claim to improve your overall physical condition. They may, in some cases, help to reduce or alleviate some of the painful complications of diabetes, such as those affecting the nerves or circulation.

Physical therapies can also promote a sense of well-being, so there is some overlap with the therapies that help the mind and emotions. A good example of this is yoga – one of the few therapies proven to improve diabetic control in a number of studies in Britain, America and India.

These techniques help the body meet the challenges of being a diabetic, as well as providing improved relaxation skills.

All the therapies discussed in this chapter are safe and natural. If they do bring about alterations in insulin requirements, any changes to your daily dosage should be made only after discussion with your doctor. Your doctor may recommend some of these therapies in combination with your conventional treatment.

Therapies which might help you to manage your diabetes more effectively are:

- acupuncture
- acupressure (shiatsu)
- aromatherapy
- homoeopathy

- massage
- reflexology
- traditional Oriental (Chinese and Indian) medicine
- yoga

Acupuncture

As most people know, acupuncture is an ancient system of healing that forms a central part of the traditional medicine of China. But it is now rapidly becoming a part of both the natural therapy and conventional medicine menu in the West also.

The aim of acupuncture is to restore the balance in the body of *qi* (pronounced 'chee', and meaning 'energy' or 'life force') and so to boost parts of the body considered 'weak'. Traditional Chinese medicine views the body as a balance between the *yin* (negative) force and the *yang* (positive), the two complementary qualities of this energy force.

According to Chinese belief *qi* flows through *meridians*, or channels beneath the skin, that run like a network throughout the body. Disharmony and disease follow when these energy lines become blocked, disturbing the flow of life force. The reason for the very fine needles inserted in acupuncture is to unblock the energy lines to restore the balance.

The needles – normally of stainless steel, silver or gold – are usually left in place for 20–30 minutes. Alternatively they may be agitated by the therapist for greater effect. Some practitioners now do this using a mild electric current instead, a technique known as *electro-acupuncture*.

People who have had acupuncture say it is quite painless and induces a pleasant feeling of deep relaxation.

A variation is a technique known as *moxibustion*. This involves the smouldering of herbs, or *moxa*, placed on

June's story

'I was diagnosed as a Type II diabetic seven years ago. Before diagnosis I had never felt so strange in my life. I thought I was dying. Driving to work, sweat would pour down my face. I could not go on a 10-mile car journey without plenty to drink. At night I would stand at the sink and drink glass after glass of water.

'As soon as I was diagnosed I was put on tablets. Then I lived abroad for two years in Tenerife and I had a far less stressed lifestyle. I came off the tablets.

'A year ago I was introduced to acupuncture by my daughter, and it has helped me enormously. The benefit I get out of it is the feeling afterwards. I have no more worries. If I don't have my acupuncture for two weeks then I begin to feel I really need it. I miss it.

'What happens is needles are placed in my feet and ankles, the room is warm, the lights are dimmed, and I just seem to drift off into a dream-like state.

'Since I have been having acupuncture, my diabetes is much better controlled. I only had one upset in 1994 when a close friend died, literally next to me, from a heart attack. My blood sugar levels went shooting up.

'But after having acupuncture I began to feel better, and the diabetes calmed down.

'On occasions I have had a needle placed on the top of my head. The acupuncturist describes me on these occasions as just like a pressure-cooker needing to let off steam. It really helps.'

the end either of a needle or 'moxa stick' held near to the acupuncture point.

Acupuncture and moxibustion are not known as treatments for diabetes but there are practitioners who use them to treat the condition. Dr Nicholas Haines, the founder of the Northern Acupuncture College in England, claims they are useful for the complications of the disease and for tackling the 'hidden progression' of diabetes, but there is little research in the West to confirm this idea.

There is no set number of treatments but some Type II diabetics say it has helped them. You should notice a difference after about five sessions. There is no evidence of it helping Type I diabetics.

Acupressure

Acupressure has been described as acupuncture without needles, and there is even a theory it may have been in use in the Orient before acupuncture. There are a number of variations but perhaps the best known is *shiatsu*.

Shiatsu is a Japanese word meaning 'finger pressure' and just like acupuncture the principles are based on the flow of *qi* or 'life force' through specific channels in the body.

Practitioners use thumbs, fingers, elbows, and even knees and feet to apply pressure and stimulate the 'energy lines'.

Physically this has the effect of stimulating circulation and, possibly, the hormonal system. The therapy also encourages deep relaxation and is therefore useful in dealing with stress. Practitioners may also give advice on diet, exercise and lifestyle.

Aromatherapy

Aromatherapy is believed to have been around for some 5,000 years. Certainly the medicinal use of plants and oils was known about in ancient Egypt and is mentioned in very early Chinese writings.

The art was revived this century by French physician Dr Jean Valnet who used essential oils derived from plants, bark, petals, wood and spices to treat diabetes, amongst other chronic diseases, after the First World War. He was so successful that other doctors took up his work and today aromatherapy is an accepted part of the conventional medical scene in France.

The therapy moved into other European countries after the Second World War, particularly Britain, and it is now one of the fastest-growing natural therapies around.

Aromatherapy has been found to be highly effective in treating stress and nervous problems, and may play a part in healing physical wounds. This is helpful for diabetics with leg or foot ulcers, or wounds which are infected and proving hard to heal.

There are over 40 different oils to choose from and you can either consult a skilled therapist or buy oils and use them at home yourself. The normal method of applying them is by massage but they can be inhaled, put in the bath or used as a compress. Foot and hand baths are particularly soothing and effective for circulatory problems.

Aromatherapy for diabetes is best seen as a complement to any conventional treatments and can support the body in its fight against the disease.

Massaging essential oils into the body is therapeutic for circulatory disorders, a complication of diabetes. It is also helpful for lowering blood pressure and releasing tension. One aromatherapist described the overall effect of massage and oils as 'semi-hypnotic'. It is certainly a deeply relaxing and even sensual experience.

Inhaling essential oils stimulates the part of the brain connected to hormone control, instinctive behaviour and strong emotions.

Oils that may help diabetes include *sage* (for circulation), *orange blossom* (stress), *lemon* (poor circulation and high blood pressure), *frankincense* (skin problems and stress), and *lavender* (calming and soothing).

The antiseptic qualities of *tea-tree oil* have also found to be helpful in treating some of the painful foot ulcerations suffered as a complication of diabetes.

A bath oil containing *camphor, eucalyptus, geranium, juniper, lemon* and *rosemary* may help balance secretions from the pancreas. A back massage, using a vegetable oil base, and using six to eight drops of the above ingredients, is also said to help.

You can buy oils over the counter in many shops and practise at home with your partner. But quality varies enormously and it is true you get what you pay for. Some cheap oils can be therapeutically almost useless.

With a condition like diabetes it is best to try to seek out a specialist in *medical* aromatherapy who will know a lot more than therapists who use the oils as beauty treatments rather than remedies.

A word of caution   Oils should *always* be diluted according to the recommendations and *never* taken by mouth except under the instructions of a medically-qualified specialist. Even diluted essential oils are powerful and should *never* be used on small children or pregnant women.

Homoeopathy

Homoeopathic treatments follow the 200-year-old principle established by a German doctor, Samuel

Hahnemann, that 'like cures like'. Homoeopathic medicines are made from a variety of sources – animal vegetable and mineral.

Very small amounts form a solution which is diluted and vigorously shaken. Homoeopaths believe that the more dilute the solution and the more it is shaken, the more potent the result – which is why most doctors find it hard to accept. The principle is the very opposite of the science they were taught at college.

Some homoeopaths claim that diabetics can be treated with homoeopathic remedies, but bear in mind that nothing will restore insulin-producing cells in the body if you are a Type I diabetic.

Homoeopathic treatments will usually be prescribed for general overall improvement in health, or for specific complications of the disease such as heart, nerve and kidney disease. Examples are:

- For general constitution: *nat sulph, silicea, argent nit*, and *phosphoric AC*.
- For neuralgia: *aconite 30C* (when nerves flare up after exposure to cold), *lachesis 6C* (pain worse after sleep), *mag phos 6C* (pain eases by heat or pressure over painful area), *arsenicum 6C* (pain when patient feels exhausted or chilly).
- For retinopathy: *arnica 30C* (as soon as 'floaters' are seen), *conium 6C* (if arnica does not help within 24 hours) or *lachesis 6C* (to help prevent further leaking of tiny blood vessels). But bear in mind this condition can be an emergency so you should seek proper medical help. A doctor qualified in homoeopathy is ideal.

In fact, in general, although remedies are available over the counter, you should always consult a qualified practitioner when taking homoeopathic remedies for a serious condition such as diabetes. They tend not to work unless tailored to your individual needs. If you are taking conventional medicines as well, always consult your family doctor in any case.

Massage

Massage is one of the oldest and most influential touch therapies and is a very effective way of treating or managing stress. It can quickly restore an overall sense of bodily well-being and energy as well as soothe and calm the mind and restore self-confidence.

The range of techniques is wide, from the vigorous Swedish style to soft touch methods such as shiatsu where you are hardly aware of the touch at all. Somewhere between falls 'holistic massage' – which claims to treat the spiritual as well as physical 'whole person' but is really only gentle massage under a fashionable new name.

On a physical level, massage encourages the body to deal with waste products effectively and aids circulation.

Reflexology

Reflexology is based on the idea that 'zones', or areas, on the feet (and sometimes the hands) correspond to different organs and parts of the body. For example, the zone of the pancreas is in the arch of the foot.

In simple terms reflexologists use the feet as 'maps' of the body and use information they find there to assess a person's state of health.

The therapy borrows largely from the principles behind Chinese medicine. So therapists believe that by applying pressure to these areas on the feet or hands, energy channels in the body are unblocked and restored.

There is no scientific evidence for this as yet, which is why so many doctors find it hard to accept. But the therapy's benefits have been so evident in so many cases –

particularly for stress – that nurses especially are now using it widely in hospitals in many countries.

Certainly reflexology offers a sense of wellbeing and will help improve circulation. It may also be useful for relieving painful nerve problems, a common complication for diabetics.

A modern 'hi-tech' version, which is called *Vacuflex* and is becoming popular in some countries, claims to achieve the same results more quickly and better by using special felt boots and suction pads operated by a vacuum pump, although there is no proof that it is beneficial for diabetics.

Traditional Oriental medicines

Two of the oldest medical systems known to humankind claim to have much to offer the modern diabetic. They are:

- Traditional Chinese Medicine (TCM) and
- Ayurvedic medicine (traditional Indian medicine)

Traditional Chinese Medicine

TCM combines the use of herbs and acupuncture as part of an elaborate philosophy that sees disease in a completely different way from Western medicine. It involves a complex diagnostic system that includes examining tongue, ears, face, hands and feet, and may include counselling and dietary advice.

The underlying purpose of the method is to restore the *yin/yang* balance – the balance between the physical and the emotional.

A herbalist may have access to several hundred different herbs which can be formulated into teas, powders, creams, lotions and pills. A standard preparation for diabetes is known as 'Eight Flavour' tea which combines eight different herbs in tablet or powder form.

Researchers at Aston University in central England who have been investigating natural remedies for diabetes (see *Chapter 9*) found that *Xiaoke* tea, an infusion of dried leaves, has some impact on lowering glucose levels.

Diabetes may be considered to be a kidney and spleen imbalance and herbs would be prescribed to restore the *yin* and the *yang*, to nourish 'weak' organs, and generally strengthen the body.

Ayurvedic medicine

Ayurvedic medicine is the main form of traditional medicine in India and has been described as one the 'most ancient and complete systems of natural healthcare in the world'. It has a growing following in the West.

The system is part of a wider philosophy of life known as *Ayurveda* – meaning 'science of life' – and involves 20 different approaches to health through mind, body, behaviour and environment. Emphasis is placed on diet and nutrition, lifestyle, environment and emotions.

Herbal and mineral preparations are used (there are some 8,000 different herbal medicines in this system) and there is an emphasis on prevention and correcting imbalances in the body before disease takes hold.

Apart from prescribed herbs, treatment relies heavily on changing lifestyle and diet – both factors in conventional diabetic care also.

Importance is placed on content and preparation of food, and the belief is that certain foods can reduce anxiety while others increase energy levels.

Yoga

Yoga is a system of spiritual, mental and physical training that originates from India, where a number of research and learning centres exist for it. The word is taken from the Sanskrit and means 'union' (the English word 'yoke' comes from it).

The study of true yoga incorporates elements such as meditation, and requires a certain amount of spiritual commitment. The yoga we know most about in the West is only one aspect of yoga, the physical aspect more accurately called *Hatha Yoga*. This is the umbrella term for the postures and exercises called *asanas*, which should really be practised together with breathing and relaxation exercises.

Yoga in the West is usually taught and practised in groups but work on your own at home is also possible.

Yoga therapy promotes the body's own natural healing resources by using the ancient physical and mental techniques directed at specific ailments and conditions. The approach is holistic: a combination of simple postures, breathing and relaxation exercises are taught, to promote better mental, physical and emotional functions.

Researchers who have looked at the effect of yoga on diabetics feel that a major benefit is the way yoga encourages body control and body awareness.

As a diabetic you may sometimes feel your body controls you because of the need to monitor and regulate food and medication. This can lead to negative feelings and lowered self-esteem.

In Britain the Yoga Biomedical Trust in London has organized research into the effect of yoga on diabetes, and runs special classes and groups specifically for diabetics.

Six years ago the trust was involved in the first British research work on yoga and diabetes at the Royal Free Hospital in London. Type II diabetics found that after 3 months of yoga sessions five times a week they showed reductions in their blood glucose levels, blood pressure and weight.

Trust director Dr Robin Monro believes that yoga is a

positive influence for both types of diabetics and its prolonged use in Type II may eliminate the need to take oral
tablets or insulin altogether.

He claims that in India there is even greater evidence of
the effectiveness of yoga in both Types I and II diabetes,
particularly from work in research centres in Bombay and
Bangalore – although most Indian research is not carried
out in the same way as clinical trials in the West.

'Indian diabetics have less rigid control than they do
in the West, so in some ways the results of working with
diabetics and yoga in India shows even more promise
and better results', he says.

Yoga and diabetes research

A total of 149 Type II diabetics underwent 40 days of yoga
therapy at the Central Research Institute for Yoga in Delhi.
Of the total, 104 patients showed a 'fair to good' response
with a 'significant' reduction in hyperglycaemia and a
decrease in the need for glucose-lowering tablets.

The report, published in the *Diabetes Research and
Clinical Practice Journal* in 1993, concluded that 'yoga, a
simple and economical therapy, may be considered a beneficial adjuvant for non-insulin-dependent patients'.

Yoga exercises for diabetics
The benefits of yoga come through regular and frequent
practice. Set aside a time each day for yoga, maybe
before breakfast or before your evening meal. Before you
start, choose some breathing and stretching exercises.

The exercises in *figure 10* have been shown to be of
particular benefit for diabetes but make sure you incor-
porate them into a balanced yoga programme, and seek
advice from a specialist yoga teacher if you are unsure
about the postures. Also seek advice and ask for a modi-
fied programme if you are pregnant, or if you have
hypertension or heart disease.

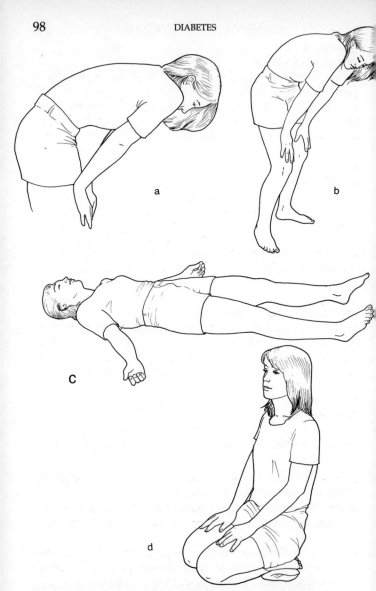

Fig. 10 Four simple yoga exercises to do at home
From *Yoga for Common Ailments* (see *Further Reading*)

Exercise A
The abdominal lock
Bend forward and exhale completely through your mouth. Then close your throat so no air can enter. Expand your chest as though inhaling and suck in your abdomen forming a deep hollow. Try to relax the muscles. Hold until you need a breath, then release and inhale slowly.

Exercise B
Abdominal pumping
Lean forward and exhale completely through your mouth. Close your throat so air cannot enter your lungs. Expand your chest as if inhaling and suck your abdomen up into the chest. Then with your lungs empty, relax your muscles so the abdomen comes out. Suck in the abdomen and pump it in and out until you need to inhale, then breathe normally.

Exercise C
The corpse pose (for relaxation)
Lie on your back on a flat, firm surface. Reduce the gap beneath your lower back by lifting your knees to your chest, then slide your feet along the floor as you lower your legs. Spread your arms out beside you, palms upwards. Relax.

Exercise D
Sectional or yoga breathing
This should come naturally as part of a daily session. Breathe slowly and evenly and stop for a moment after exhaling or inhaling.

- Inhale by letting your abdomen bulge and then exhale by drawing in slowly and continuously.
- Hold your shoulders and abdomen still as you inhale by expanding your lower rib cage. Exhale by slowly releasing your ribs.
- Hold your abdomen slightly in and your lower rib cage stationary. Breathe in and out by allowing your collar bones, upper chest and shoulders to move up and down.

Patricia's story

'I am a grandmother of seven and have had non-insulin-dependent diabetes for 20 years. I don't take tablets or insulin and the only "treatment" I have is yoga. I travel up to London for sessions of yoga therapy designed specifically for diabetics. Yoga gives me a feeling of deep calm and tranquillity.

'Over the past six months I have done more advanced techniques and my blood sugar levels have dropped by three points. Yoga is not just a good form of exercise, it's a wonderful way of life.'

Summary

No physical therapies hold the promise of a cure. What they can do, however, is help you feel more positive about yourself and encourage you to have a more positive approach to life. They can also:

- strengthen your body through gentle exercise
- influence associated problems such as nerve damage and circulation problems
- relieve stress
- improve glucose control

Physical treatments also include eating and drinking and in the next chapter we'll look specifically at the many ways in which food, diet and nutrition can help diabetics.

CHAPTER 9

Eating and diabetes

How different foods can help diabetes

Food is a fundamental factor, a cornerstone if you like, in the day-by-day management of diabetes. Diabetic symptoms can improve or deteriorate because of what you eat and drink.

Food scientists and researchers are currently discovering more about the physical and chemical properties of food. The active components of food are the focus of research into how food might be developed with certain 'desired' properties – such as an ability to lower blood glucose levels in diabetics, for example.

Certain foods have the ability to influence the course of the diabetes by:

- lowering blood glucose levels
- encouraging the uptake of insulin
- altering the levels of lipids in the blood
- improving overall health
- playing a part in slowing down complications such as heart and kidney disease

But this is such a new area that at present the British Diabetic Association and the American Dietetic Association recommend only that diabetics follow a healthy 'normal' diet.

For diabetics a 'normal healthy diet', as discussed in *Chapter 4*, means selecting a wide range of foods but concentrating on low saturated fat, complex carbohydrate foods such as baked potatoes, wholemeal bread and pasta, reducing salt intake and eating medium amounts of protein from a variety of sources.

There is nothing wrong with this advice. At present 30 per cent of Type II diabetics are treated by diet – meaning a healthier as well as a weight-reducing diet – and a further 50 per cent are treated with a combination of drugs to lower blood sugar levels and diet. The rest require insulin to meet their body's demands. But adopting a healthier diet is also encouraged.

A 'good' diet also plays a role in managing impaired glucose tolerance and is just as important for Type I diabetics.

But there is more: scientists are now discovering almost every month there are *particular* elements of food that are naturally therapeutic. Incorporating some of them into your diet could help your diabetes even more than just eating healthily. These new 'designer'-type foods are known as *functional foods* and were created by scientists in a laboratory for diabetics.

Functional foods

Functional foods are a new type of food with huge potential to be of benefit to diabetics, especially in helping them with glucose control. The first such foods appeared on supermarket shelves in Europe during 1995 and could revolutionize eating for diabetics.

The name 'functional' means both nutritious and therapeutic. Functional foods contain specific ingredients that could help diabetics achieve dietary goals much more easily than with 'ordinary' foods.

The idea of designer food started in Japan. The Japanese consider foods containing physiologically active ingredients and delivering health benefits to the population at large as the food of the future.

The first of these new foods are of particular benefit to diabetics. They are:

- guar bread rolls
- oatbran-enriched breakfast cereal

Guar bread rolls are derived from guar gum and have been created by food scientists in Britain with a special interest in Type II diabetes and metabolism (see box). If successful they could be followed by biscuits, crackers and breakfast cereals.

The guar in the bread effectively reduces the rise in blood glucose after eating when compared to a meal not containing guar. Eating the guar bread rolls produces a rise in blood glucose, but not as high as the rise which occurs after eating ordinary bread.

The guar gum story

Guar gum looks an innocuous little bean but it holds tremendous potential for diabetics. The Indian cluster bean or *Cyamopsis tetragonoloba* is a green sickle-shaped bean traditionally used in India and Pakistan (see *figure 11*). Guar gum is extracted from the seed's endosperm or 'energy store'.

The earliest work with guar was done in the 1960s, when it was recognized that guar and other *polysaccharides* had the ability to lower blood cholesterol levels in animals. But it was not until the 1970s that it was recognized that guar could also affect rises in both blood glucose and insulin after meals in humans, including those with diabetes.

Early pioneering work by Professor David Jenkins of the University of Toronto, Canada, and UK research by Dr Tony Leeds and Dr Peter Ellis of King's College, London, at the Central Middlesex Hospital in London and the Radcliffe Infirmary, Oxford, with Type II diabetics was so successful that guar gum was tested in drinks or sprinkled in granule form over food.

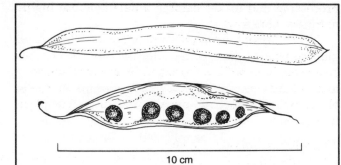

Fig. 11 Seeds of the Indian cluster bean – source of guar gum

Although the results looked good, the drinks were thick and very unpalatable. It was then that work started on the new type of processing leading to the launch of the new guar bread rolls.

It is hoped the new rolls will be far more palatable and acceptable as an alternative to wholemeal bread. They should be useful not only for diabetics but also those at risk of heart disease.

The oatbran story

Studies in Canada by Dr Peter Wood in 1993 showed that oat gum and oatbran used in porridge meals given to Type II diabetics lowered blood glucose levels. The Swiss company Nestlé are currently testing a new oatbran, rolled oat and wheat breakfast cereal and this could be on the market by 1996 aimed specifically at diabetics.

Nestlé claim the new food will have the same taste and texture as other oat cereals but with a far more beneficial effect on both cholesterol and glucose levels.

Oatbran-enriched cereals contain 50 per cent more oatbran fibre than other cereals and are thought to have great potential in lowering blood glucose levels in diabetics. The new cereal involves a pioneering type of processing that makes oatbran a palatable but highly nutritious fibre-food.

This ability of food to play a part in controlling blood glucose levels falls directly into line with the targets being sought in both America and Britain for diabetics – to prevent as far as possible the high and low swings in blood glucose levels in order to avoid future complications like heart and kidney disease.

The future of functional foods

Clinicians and dietitians recognize that one of the problems facing Type II diabetics is the 'healthy' diet.

Although foods such as bread, rice and potatoes are actively encouraged in a good diet, many of these foods actually have a *high Glycaemic Index*, which means that eating them causes higher rises in the levels of blood glucose than other foods such as beans, legumes and pasta.

One of the long-term aims of leading researchers into the problem in Britain, America, Japan and Sweden is to try to convert common high glycaemic foods into low glycaemic foods by adding ingredients such as guar and without losing their palatability.

Dr Peter Ellis and research colleagues at King's College, London, are looking at other 'natural' alternatives, such as plant polysaccharides, with similar glucose-lowering effects, including two different Nigerian plants.

Soups containing extracts from *Detarium senegalense*, a Nigerian legume, and *Cissus rotundifolia*, a shrub, have been found significantly to reduce blood sugar and insulin rises in healthy human subjects. In 1995 these beans were undergoing tests with diabetic patients at St Thomas's in London.

Dr Ellis says that the relationship between the physical and chemical properties in the food people eat and their nutrition and health is still poorly understood –

even though experts are beginning to understand what constitutes a healthy diet.

'It is far more complex than just eating well', he says. 'Understanding how nutrients in food are digested and then absorbed is important for determining the health benefits of particular diets.

'We still need to know much more about the way food is handled by our bodies and its metabolic effect.'

Researching the way food behaves in the gastro-intestinal tract and its effect on metabolism is attracting interest from a number of influential quarters.

A major symposium on functional foods held in London in March 1995 brought together food scientists, nutritionists and food manufacturers to examine this new blurring of lines between food and pharmaceuticals.

The participants were told that diabetes, heart disease and cancer were the targets for a new type of food with the ability to treat symptoms. In the future, it is hoped, patients will have a wider selection of foods that will help to improve glycaemic control.

Other foods that can help

Over 15 years ago Dr Brian Leatherdale, a consultant at Dudley Road Hospital in central England, began to see a large number of Asian diabetics who complained they could not keep their diabetes under control. They insisted it was because they had difficulty getting hold of a traditional plant called *karela* used in India to treat diabetes.

The stories about karela kept cropping up, so Dr Leatherdale decided to investigate – and in 1981 he published the results of a clinical trial that proved that feeding the fried karela fruits to Type II diabetics produced a 'small but significant improvement in glucose tolerance'.

A further test involving a water-soluble extract of the fruit 'significantly reduced' blood glucose concentrations during an oral glucose tolerance test.

Karela (*Momordica charantia*), otherwise known as 'bitter gourd', grows as a fruit in Asia and Central and South America (see *figure 12*). In Asia it is used as a vegetable in curries, soups and stews. Cultivated varieties look rather like large gherkins and have a bitter taste which it takes time to acquire.

In Central America wild karela (which has fruits much smaller than gherkins) is made into a tea called *cerasee* and is also used as an anti-diabetic medication.

The discovery that karela could influence diabetes in some patients led researchers from Aston University, also in central England, to question whether other plants too might have this anti-diabetic power.

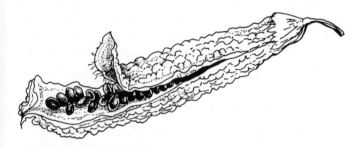

Fig. 12 The karela plant

Dr Caroline Day, a British diabetes research specialist, began a search which has so far lasted more than ten years and has resulted in the most comprehensive record of traditional remedies for diabetes to be found anywhere in the world.

Dr Day has so far collected information on about 700 different plants, herbs, vegetables and fruits with some apparent anti-diabetic quality. Most are from Asia, South America, China and Africa. The World Health

Organization has now officially recommended that traditional methods of treatment for diabetes should be further investigated.

The active property in such plants might be as simple as fibre which slows the absorption of glucose into the system (rather like guar gum). But plants such as karela, she has discovered, have other natural chemicals which play an important part in helping to control diabetes amongst its Asian followers.

Indeed, Dr Day and other researchers have now identified as many as five or six active ingredients in karela alone. However one of the stumbling blocks for making these natural chemicals more widely available is the fact that in large or concentrated doses they become toxic.

The team are isolating and investigating the natural chemicals in other plants in the hope that one day a safe, non-toxic plant chemical can be found and used as a model for a new, more natural drug to control diabetes.

Amongst the plants which have been so far investigated are the leaves of eucalyptus, juniper berries, blackber-

---

Common plants with anti-diabetic properties

The following plants contain either a natural plant chemical which plays a part in lowering blood glucose levels or high amounts of fibre which effectively slow absorption of glucose into the blood stream:

- leeks
- onions
- garlic
- fenugreek seeds
- karela
- common edible mushrooms

- coriander seeds
- juniper berries
- cabbage
- lettuce
- potatoes
- turnips

The advice from nutritionists is that there is no harm in incorporating these foods into a well-balanced daily diet, but never eat them in large amounts on their own.

ry leaves, a Mexican cactus called *Opuntia streptacantha* and infusions of alfalfa from South Africa which contain high levels of manganese. Alfalfa also has a high vitamin K content and a synthetic version of this vitamin can mimic certain effects of insulin.

A double-blind trial using ivy gourd (*Coccina indica*) has shown promising results, with a 20 per cent drop in glucose concentration amongst Type II diabetics who were prescribed an infusion of leaves.

Dr Day suggests there is nothing wrong with including vegetables like karela in the diet as long as it is in moderation and blood glucose levels are monitored if you decide to eat it regularly.

Monounsaturated fats

Research has shown that both Type I and Type II diabetics might benefit from a diet high in monounsaturated fats found in such foods as olive oil and avocados, macadamia nuts and almonds.

Monounsaturated fats appear to have a very beneficial influence on diabetes by lowering both blood glucose and harmful blood fat levels in the blood stream while maintaining the good (HDL) cholesterol levels.

Studies in New Zealand and Australia have come out in favour of a Mediterranean-style olive oil-rich diet against diets high in complex carbohydrate.

The only drawback to the 'olive oil' diet is getting the calorie level correct if you are overweight. A first positive step would be to learn to replace saturated fat, such as butter and margarine, with items such as peanut or olive oil.

A dietician could advise you on how to juggle your calories so that you don't end up eating too much of a good thing!

Vegetarian diets

There is some evidence that a vegetarian diet might slow down diabetic kidney disease.

Food supplements

Food supplements are concentrated doses of vitamins, minerals, amino acids, essential fatty acids and enzymes in tablet, capsule or, sometimes, powder form, used to prevent, treat and overcome illness.

They are normally prescribed in therapeutic doses by practitioners such as *nutritional therapists, naturopaths* and, more rarely, *medical herbalists.*

Essential fatty acids

Essential fatty acids are the outstanding success story of those food supplements said to be effective for diabetes. An essential fatty acid is a substance that cannot be manufactured by the body and so, like vitamins, needs to be included in the diet.

The best known is evening primrose oil (see *figure 13*). Evening primrose oil (EPO) has proved to be a breakthrough in the natural treatment of two serious diabetic complications: diabetic neuropathy and retinopathy. The active ingredient in EPO is *gamma linoleic acid* (GLA).

GLA is one of a number, or family, of essential fatty acids (EFAs) that are vital components of the structure of all cell membranes. EFAs are converted in the body into *prostaglandins*, vital chemicals that regulate many body functions such as the heart, kidneys, liver, lungs, brain, nerves, skin and immune system.

Scientists have recognized that diabetics have a problem metabolizing EFAs and so have much reduced levels of essential fatty acids circulating in their blood. In particular diabetes 'blocks' the conversion in the body of the essential fatty acid linoleic acid to GLA. By taking supplements of GLA it is technically possible, therefore, to bypass this blockage and supply 'pure' GLA to the body via capsules.

The seed of the evening primrose plant contains large amounts of GLA but it still takes 5,000 tiny seeds to yield the oil for just one 500 milligram capsule.

Studies into GLA – which is also found in large quantities in borage (starflower), blackcurrant seed oil and oils from fungi or moulds as well as in human breast-milk and polyunsaturated vegetable oils – and its role in the prevention of disease over the last 20 years in Britain, The Netherlands, Japan, America and Switzerland have all shown good results in diabetes.

For example, research involving 133 patients in the UK and Finland with diabetic nerve damage showed that those who took large doses of daily supplements (up to 12 times the recommended daily amount) improved, while those who did not deteriorated.

Trials in Canada have also shown conclusively that EPO can stop, and even reverse, diabetic neuropathy.

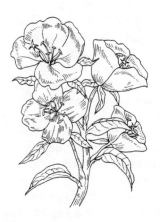

Fig. 13 The evening primrose flower

Scientists in France and Australia, too, have come up with evidence that diabetics cannot produce GLA normally – and this, they believe, may be the root cause of some of the long-term complications of diabetes.

Yet more studies have shown that GLAs such as EPO can help slow down the development of eye damage from diabetes. Another beneficial spin-off is the way GLA influences the levels of harmful fats circulating in the blood.

EPO is available on prescription or over the counter in pharmacies and healthfood stores in most countries. But it is worth pointing out that some of the studies organized under strict scientific control involved very high doses – up to 6 grams a day (12x500 milligram capsules) – to be effective.

For further information or help consult a nutritional therapist or a company producing EPO (such as, in Britain, Efamol).

Sheila's story

Sheila Black, a former actress and distinguished economist and journalist, was diagnosed as a Type II diabetic 15 years ago at the age of 60.

Although she controlled her diabetes well, she developed the most painful complication of diabetes: diabetic neuropathy. She was told there was no conventional cure.

'I can stand pain. A couple of times in my life I have had to and coped pretty well. But the deep, all over, burning, consistent, permanent pain of diabetic neuropathy was unbearable.

'To me, only death could bring relief. I told my family not to grieve if they found I had managed to end it all in some foolproof way.

'It was nothing to do with my love for them, only with the impossibility of living with incessant, deep pain, with no sleep and, I thought, no hope.'

Sheila's doctor explained that despite good diabetic control she had damaged nerve-endings that were sending distorted and painful messages around her body, especially to the thighs, middle and legs.

The pain did not react to painkillers and she was told there was no known conventional cure, although a gel and sleeping tablets did help manage the problem.

One day she was advised to try oil of evening primrose and her doctor did not stand in her way.

'I started taking Efamol evening primrose oil in large daily doses [6 grams a day] in the November. By February, on the night of a reunion dinner, I found myself thinking that I would have liked to be there and might have managed it after all.

'This was a first. I hadn't wanted to do anything for months. It was a landmark because, after that, I began to do things I just could never have faced earlier. I still couldn't drive because my legs and arms buckled when pain shot through them. But gradually, very gradually but very obviously, the pains lessened – both in degree and in frequency. I could sit without jumping with pain and without stiffening. It was getting better.

'Through March it was marked, and in April I took two train journeys to visit my daughter.

'When my birthday came in May I gave a small party, staying up late. And then I realized it was exactly six months since I had started taking the evening primrose oil.

'Progress since then has been exactly that – progressive. My nerves, my whole body, feel regenerated.'

Minerals and trace elements

There are four minerals which appear to play an important role in diabetes:

- zinc (required to assist in the release of insulin from the 'beta' cells in the pancreas)
- chromium (plays an important role in insulin production and in helping insulin to control blood glucose)
- magnesium (a lack might contribute to insulin resistance among Type II diabetics)
- vanadium

Although it is known that these minerals are involved in metabolic control it has not yet been established whether supplementing your diet with these minerals will have any real effect upon your diabetes and experts are divided over the issue.

Zinc

The body can't store zinc so there is a good argument that supplementing with zinc tablets might be beneficial. Without zinc, insulin cannot be released to work on glucose in the blood, and deficiencies have been reported among Type II diabetics who become insulin resistant.

Zinc, found naturally in liver, eggs and fish, also helps heal wounds caused by the complications of diabetes.

Chromium

Highly-refined foods are low in chromium and there is some evidence that people who eat a lot of sugary foods have low levels of chromium. Richard Anderson, a biochemist at the US Department of Agriculture's Human Nutrition Centre, says: 'There is overwhelming evidence that chromium does regulate and improve insulin activity. In the presence of sufficient amounts of biologically active chromium, much lower amounts of insulin are required' (Juvenile Diabetes Federation 1995 Research Journal *Countdown*).

However Professor Anthony Diplock, one of Britain's leading antioxidant researchers, says: 'There is no evidence that diabetics are lacking in chromium if they eat a reasonable diet.'

Scientists hope to find out more through following a one-year research project that will involve giving Type II diabetics chromium-rich brewer's yeast supplements every day, and monitoring their metabolic reactions. The study is being organized by trace element experts at the Food Research Institute in Norwich, UK.

You can buy chromium supplements from healthfood stores and the best natural sources are foods such as cereals, legumes (peas and beans), nuts and brewer's yeast.

Magnesium

Researchers in America are looking at the importance of magnesium in the diet of diabetics. A lack of magnesium may play a role in insulin resistance, carbohydrate intolerance and hypertension (high blood pressure). There is a case for supplementing with magnesium if you have poor glycaemic control.

Vanadium

Vanadium is a trace element being looked at keenly for its possible use in diabetes.

Vitamins

Despite some evidence that supplementing a healthy diet with the well-known cure-all, vitamin C, can actually be harmful for diabetics in too high doses, there is a wealth of evidence in the other direction: that the right vitamins in the right doses for the right condition can be very beneficial.

Vitamin E, for example, is beneficial for overall health and for insulin uptake, especially amongst older Type II diabetics.

Low levels of vitamin E, the most powerful 'antioxidant' (anti-ageing) vitamin known, have been found to be an important risk factor in the development of heart disease, though its role in diabetes is only just being looked at.

A study in Italy in 1993 showed that daily vitamin E supplements produced a small but significant improvement in the metabolic control of Type II diabetes (but it also pointed out that more work needs to be done to check the safety of high doses of vitamin E supplements for diabetics).

Note Heart disease in diabetics is caused by different factors to those in the rest of the population so treatments appropriate for cardiovascular patients will not necessarily be appropriate for diabetics with heart disease complications.

Naturopathic medicine

Practitioners of naturopathic medicine are known as 'naturopaths'. Naturopaths specialize in a range of natural therapies and are the nearest thing to a 'general practitioner' of natural medicine.

A skilled naturopath may use osteopathy – a system of manipulating the bones and muscles of the body, especially the back, to restore physical and mental wellbeing – acupuncture, hydrotherapy, homoeopathy, herbs and food supplements as well as psychotherapy and counselling.

Like all other natural therapists, naturopaths view disease as an imbalance in the body and will try to restore the body's own healing powers. They will want to try to find out which factors made you vulnerable to 'dis-ease', as they put it.

There is an emphasis on good nutrition, a healthy lifestyle and positive thinking. Exercise and weight loss are also an important part of overall treatment.

So the typical naturopath is likely to take many of the elements discussed already in this book together to treat your diabetes. For Type II diabetics the major emphasis will be on improving diet and lifestyle and on relaxation skills. For Type I diabetics the main focus will be on boosting health, and improving general overall well-being.

Naturopaths are commonest in America, South Africa, Australia, New Zealand, Germany and Israel where their training covers much the same ground as conventional medical doctors and where they are sometimes recognized as having equal status. Many work alongside family practitioners in those countries as a result.

Medical herbalism

Medical herbalists use plants to treat and prevent disease. They may use some of the plants mentioned already to treat your diabetes: there are plenty of plants that can be used to lower blood glucose levels, for example, and medical herbalists might also suggest others to improve the function of the liver and pancreas.

But medical herbalism is a serious and refined therapy in which herbalists are thoroughly trained to use quite potent and, sometimes, dangerous herbs that no one untrained should even attempt.

Medical herbalists take a 'whole person' view of their patients and aim to restore the balance of the body by enabling it to mobilize its own healing powers. Treatment might also include advice about diet and lifestyle.

If you are a Type I diabetic you should seek advice from your family doctor before you accept a herbal prescription – although a reputable herbalist will want to

talk to your doctor and ask about your insulin requirements.

Don't expect to be able to give up insulin – though, in
some cases, you may be able to reduce insulin doses
under the supervision of your medical herbalist and
family practitioner (or 'diabetologist'), if the herbs
improve insulin uptake.

Herbal treatments for Type II diabetics who manage
their diabetes by diet alone might include *nettle, goat's
rue, dandelion root* or *fingertree bark*. These improve the
function of the liver and pancreas and are usually prescribed as tinctures rather than teas as many such herbs
have a very bitter taste.

Summary

We have seen that a variety of practitioners and therapists can help most people with both main types of diabetes a great deal. But the next question is almost the
most important, and the hardest to answer: how do you
find a therapist you can rely on? The final chapter tells
you exactly how.

CHAPTER 10

How to find and choose a natural therapist

Tips and guidelines for finding reliable help

It is much easier now to find the right therapist than it was even a few years ago – but it is still not easy enough. The sheer variety of therapies is bewildering in itself and in many countries natural therapists are still not fully organized. There is no shortage of directories and adverts but it is difficult to assess the reliability of their information. So how do you find a therapist you can trust?

Starting the search: local sources

As we have seen, many of the natural therapies highlighted in this book have their roots in antiquity. Some have existed for as long as human beings have lived on earth, and finding a good practitioner has been a matter of tuning in to the community 'bush telegraph'. Word of mouth is still the best way to find the right practitioner.

Speak to anyone whose opinion you respect, especially if he or she is also a fellow sufferer. (You will also want to know who should be avoided, and which therapies might not help you at all.) If this does not work there are several other ways you can try:

Doctors' clinics and medical centres

If you need help urgently you must see your family doctor. It has already been explained in this book that your condition can decline quickly without the proper treatment. If you ask about natural therapies at your first appointment, be prepared to hear anything from a dire warning to a recommendation that you might try a natural therapist once your condition is stable.

Natural health centres

Your nearest natural health centre should be happy to advise you. Your first impressions will often be a good guide to the quality of service they provide. Are the staff well informed and friendly? Is the place clean and comfortable? Does the atmosphere make you feel comfortable from the moment you walk in? It should. It matters. You are bringing them your trust and your custom and both should be treated with the utmost respect.

A good centre should have plenty of information explaining the therapies and introducing the practitioners. In a well-run practice the receptionist or owner will know all about the different therapies on offer. It's a bad sign if they don't.

You may still be unsure after your first impressions whether to book in or not. If so, ask to meet the person who might be treating you, just to test the waters. This should be possible, even in a busy practice.

Don't start off by telling your full life history, but some practices do offer you this opportunity during a free consultation – usually 15 minutes – just to see whether you have come to the right place or not.

Local practitioners

Practitioners tend to know who's who in the area, even in therapies other than their own. So if you know, say, a reflexologist, but want a homoeopath, ask for a recommendation. The same applies if you know a practitioner

socially and so don't want to consult him or her profes-
sionally. Practitioners are usually happy to recommend
someone else in the same field.

Healthfood stores and alternative bookshops

The staff in these kinds of shops often have a good local
knowledge as well as an interest in the subject of natural
therapies. The shop may well have a noticeboard with
local practitioners' business cards on it. Remember,
though, the most experienced and well-established practitioners don't need this kind of advertising, so you
might miss them altogether if you don't actually check
up by asking.

Other sources of local knowledge

Don't forget that your local pharmacist often has con-
tacts with both conventional and natural therapists.

The local library or information centre may be another
good source of contact, especially for finding self-help or
support groups.

Computers (using a modem) can provide this type of
information via the Internet system and other sources
worth trying are health farms, beauty therapists and citi-
zens' advice bureaux.

Wider sources of information

If you have no luck on a local level, don't give up – there
are several more leads you can follow up at a national
level.

'Umbrella' organizations

The natural therapies are increasingly coming together
under 'umbrella' organizations that represent a therapy
or range of therapies nationally under one banner or
heading. These national umbrella organizations have
lists of registered and approved practitioners, and in the

case of the more established therapies (such as chiropractic) have their own regulatory bodies already in place.

It is better to phone than to write or fax because this should give you a good idea of how well organized the group is. You may find that the group you are contacting has several different associations under its banner. A small charge may be made for each association's register but if you can afford it get the lot and then make up your own mind.

Newspapers, magazines and local directories
Many therapists advertise. If you find local practitioners this way it's a good idea to talk to them and check them out first.

Checking professional organizations

Some organizations are genuine groups that really keep a check on their members, while others seem to spring up like weeds, apparently interested only in collecting membership fees and giving themselves credibility. This section helps you do your own weeding.

Why do professional organizations exist?
The purposes of governing bodies for natural therapies are:

- to keep up-to-date lists of their members so you can check whether someone is really on their list or not
- to protect you by making sure that their members are fully trained, licensed and insured against accident, negligence and malpractice
- to give you someone to complain to if you are unhappy with any aspect of treatment you have received, and you can't sort the matter out with your therapist
- to protect their members by giving good ethical and legal advice

- to represent their members when laws which might affect them are being made
- to work towards improvements in education for their members both before and after qualifying
- to work towards greater awareness of the benefit of each therapy in conventional medical circles
- to improve public awareness of the benefit of each therapy

Questions to ask professional organizations

A good organization will publish clear and simple information on its status and purposes along with its membership list. As they don't all do this you may find it useful to contact them again on receiving your list to ask the following:

- When was the association founded? (You may be reassured to hear it has been around for 50 years. If the association is new, however, don't reject it out of hand. Ask why it was formed – it may be innovative.)
- How many members does it have? (Size reflects public demand, as few therapists could survive in a therapy if there was no call for it. The bigger organizations generally have a better track record and greater public acceptance, but a small association may just reflect the fact that the therapy is very specialized or still in its infancy – not necessarily a bad thing.)
- When was the therapy that it represents started?
- Is it a charity or educational trust – with a proper constitution, management committee, and published accounts – or is it a private limited company? (Charities have to be non-profitmaking, work in the public interest, and be open to inspection at any time. Private companies don't.)
- Is it part of a larger network of organizations? (If so, this implies it is interested in progress by consensus with other groups, and not just in furthering its own

aims. By and large, groups that go their own way are more suspect than those that join in.)

- Does the organization have a code of ethics (upholding standards of professional behaviour) and disciplinary procedures? If so, what are they?
- How do its members gain admission to its register? Is it linked to only one school? (Beware of associations whose heads are also head of the school they represent: unbiased help may be in short supply with this type of 'one man band'.)
- Do members have to have proof of professional indemnity insurance? This should cover:
  - accidental damage to yourself or your property while you are on the practitioner's work premises
  - negligence (either the failure of the practitioner to exercise the 'duty of care' owed to you, or his falling below the standards of clinical competence demanded by his qualifications, bringing about an overall worsening of your problem)
  - malpractice (a 'falling from grace' over professional conduct, involving, for example, dishonesty, sexual misconduct or breach of confidence – your personal details should *never* be discussed with a third person without your permission)

Checking training and qualifications

If you have reassured yourself so far but are still puzzled by what the training actually involves, ask a few more questions:

- How long is the training?
- Is it full- or part-time?
- If it is part-time but shorter than a full-time course leading to the same qualifications, does the time spent at lectures and in clinic add up to the same as a full-

time course overall? (In other words, is it a short cut?)
- Does it include seeing patients under supervision at a college clinic and in real practices?
- What do the initials after the therapist's name mean? Do they denote simply membership of an organization or do they indicate in-depth study?
- Are the qualifications recognized? If so, by whom? (This is becoming more relevant as the therapy organizations group together and start to form state-recognized registers in many countries. But the really important thing to know is if the qualifications are recognized by an independent outside assessment authority.)

Making the choice

Making the final choice is a matter of using a combination of common sense and intuition, and finding the resolution to give someone a try. Don't forget that the most important part of the whole process is your resolve to feel better, to have more control over your state of health, and hopefully to see an improvement in your condition. The next most important part is that you feel comfortable with your chosen therapist.

What is it like seeing a natural therapist?

Since most natural therapists, even in those countries with state health systems, still work privately, there is no established common pattern.

Although they may all share more or less a belief in the principles outlined in Chapter 6, you are liable to come across individuals from all walks of life. You will find as much variety in dress, thinking and behaviour as there are fashions, ranging from the formal and sophisticated to the absolutely informal.

Equally, you will find their premises very different. Some will present a 'brass plaque' image, working in a clinic with a receptionist and brisk efficiency, while others will see you in their living room surrounded by plants and domestic clutter.

Remember, though, that while image may be some indication of status, it is little guarantee of ability. You are as likely to find a therapist of quality working from home as in a formal clinic.

Some characteristics, though, and probably the most important ones, are common to all natural therapists:

● They will give you far more time than you are used to with a family doctor. An initial consultation will rarely last less than an hour, and is often longer. They will ask you all about yourself so they can form a proper understanding of what makes you tick and what may be the fundamental cause(s) of your problem.
● You will have to pay for any remedies they prescribe, and they may well sell you these from their own stocks. They will also charge you for their time – though many therapists offer reduced fees for deserving cases or for people who genuinely cannot afford the full fee.

Sensible precautions

● Be sceptical of anyone who 'guarantees' you a cure. No-one (not even doctors) can do that.
● Query any attempt to book you in for a course of treatment. Your response to any natural therapy is highly individual. Of course, if the practice is a busy one, booking ahead for one or two sessions might be sensible. You should be able to cancel without penalty any sessions which prove unnecessary (but remember to give at least 24 hours' notice: some practitioners will

charge you if you don't give enough notice).

- No ethical therapist will ask for fees in advance of treatment unless for special tests or medicines – and even this is unusual. If you are asked for 'down payments' of any sort, ask exactly what they are for. If you don't like the reasons, don't pay.

- Be wary if you are not asked about your existing medication and try to give precise answers when you are asked. Be especially wary if the therapist tells you to stop or change any medically prescribed drug without talking to your doctor first. (A responsible doctor should also be happy to discuss you and your medication with a therapist.)

- Note the quality of the therapist's touch if you choose any of the relaxation or manipulation techniques such as massage, aromatherapy or osteopathy. It should never be lingering or suggestive. If, for any reason, the therapist wants to touch you on the breasts or genitals, your permission should be sought first.

- If the practitioner is of the opposite sex you are entitled to have someone of your choice in the room at the same time. Be immediately suspicious if this is not allowed. Ethical therapists will not refuse this sort of request, and if they do, it is probably best to have nothing more to do with them.

What to do if things go wrong

A practitioner is in a position of trust, and is charged with a duty of care to you at all times. It does not mean you are 'entitled' to a 'cure' just because you've paid for treatment, but if you feel you are being treated unfairly, incompetently or unethically, you have several options:

- Tackle the matter at the source of the problem, with your practitioner, either verbally or in writing.

- If he or she works in a place such as a clinic, health farm or sports centre, tell the management. They also have a duty to protect the public and should treat complaints seriously and discreetly.
- Contact the practitioner's professional organization. It should have an independent panel that investigates complaints fully and disciplines its members.
- If the offence committed is a criminal one report it to the police (but be prepared for the problem of proving one person's word against another's).
- If you feel compensation is due see a lawyer for advice.

Short of a public court case, the worst thing for a truly incompetent or unethical practitioner is bad publicity. Tell everyone about your experiences. People only need to hear the same sort of comments from a few different sources and the practitioner will probably sink without trace. Before you do so, though, try the other measures first and give yourself time to consider things calmly. Vengeance is not very healing.

A word of warning   Don't make malicious allegations without good reason. Such actions are themselves a criminal offence in most countries and you could end up in more trouble than the practitioner.

Summary

The reality is that there are few real crooks or charlatans in natural therapy. Despite the myth, there is little real money in it unless the therapist is very busy – and the chances are high that a busy therapist is a good one. Remember that no-one can know everything and no specialist qualified in any field has to get 100 per cent in the exams to be able to practise. Perfection is an ideal, not a reality, and to err is human.

It is very much for this reason that taking control of your own health is perhaps the single most important lesson underlying this book. Taking control means taking responsibility for the choices you make, and this is one of the most significant factors in successful treatment.

No-one but you can decide on a practitioner and no-one but you can determine if that practitioner is any good or not. You will know this very easily, and probably very quickly, by the way you feel about the person and the therapy, and by whether or not you get any better.

If you are not happy, the decision is yours whether to stay or move on – and continue moving until you find the right therapist for you. Don't despair if you don't find the right person first time. There is almost bound to be the right person for you somewhere and your determination to get well is the best resource you have for finding that person.

Above all, bear in mind that many people who have taken this route before you have not only been helped beyond their most optimistic dreams, but have also found a close and trusted helper who will assist in times of trouble – and who may even become a friend for life.

APPENDIX A

Useful organizations

The following listing of organizations is for information only and does not imply any endorsement, nor do the organizations listed necessarily agree with the views expressed in this book.

INTERNATIONAL

International Diabetes Federation
40 rue Washington
B – 1050 Brussels, Belgium
Tel 322 647 4414
Fax 322 640 8565

International Diabetic Athletes Association
6829 North 12th Street, Suite 205
Phoenix, AZ 85014, USA
Tel 602 230 8155

International Federation of Practitioners of Natural Therapeutics
10 Copse Close
Sheet, Petersfield
Hampshire GU31 4DL, UK
Tel 01730 266790
Fax 01730 260058

Juvenile Diabetes Foundation International
The Diabetes Research Foundation
432 Park Avenue South
New York
NY 10016 8013, USA
Tel 212 889 7575/800 223 1138

World Health Organization
Division of Noncommunicable Diseases
1211 Geneva 27
Switzerland
Tel 4122 791 3472
Fax 4122 791 0746

AUSTRALASIA

Australian Natural Therapists Association
PO Box 308
Melrose Park
South Australia 5039
Tel 618 297 9533
Fax 618 297 0003

Australian Traditional Medicine Society
PO Box 442 *or*
Suite 3, First Floor
120 Blaxland Road
Ryde
New South Wales 2112
Australia.
Tel 612 808 2825
Fax 612 809 7570

Diabetes Australia
AVA House
5/7 Phipps Place
Deakin
ACT 2600, Australia
Tel 616 285 3277
Fax 616 285 2881

Diabetes New Zealand Inc
1 Coquet Street
PO Box 54
Oamaru, 8915
South Island
New Zealand
Tel 643 434 8110
Fax 643 434 5281

New Zealand Natural Health Practitioners Accreditation Board
PO Box 37-491
Auckland, New Zealand
Tel 9 625 9966
Supported by 15 therapy organizations

NORTH AMERICA

American Academy of Medical Preventics
6151 West Century Boulevard
Suite 1114
Los Angeles
California 90045, USA
Tel 213 645 5350

American Association of Naturopathic Physicians
2800 East Madison Street,
Suite 200
Seattle
Washington 98112, USA

or
PO Box 20386
Seattle
Washington 98102, USA
Tel 206 323 7610
Fax 206 323 7612

American Diabetes Association
1660 Duke Street
Alexandria
VA 22314, USA
Tel 703 549 1500
Fax 703 836 7439

American Dietetic Association
216 West Jackson Boulevard
Suite 800
Chicago IL 60606, USA
Tel 312 899 0040
Fax 800 877 1600

American Holistic Medical Association
6728 Old McLean Village Drive
McLean, VA 22101, USA
Tel 703 556 9222

Canadian Diabetes Association
15 Toronto Street, Suite 1001
Toronto
Ontario M5C 2E3, Canada
Tel 416 363 3373
Fax 416 363 3393

Canadian Holistic Medical Association
700 Bay Street
PO Box 101, Suite 604
Toronto
Ontario M5G 1Z6, Canada
Tel 416 599 0447

L'Association du Diabete du Quebec
5635 Sherbrooke Estate
Montreal
Quebec H1N 1A3, Canada
Tel 514 259 3422
Fax 514 259 9286

SOUTHERN AFRICA

South African Diabetes Association
PO Box 3943
Cape Town 8000
South Africa
Tel 2721 461 3715
Fax 2721 462 2008

South African Homoeopaths, Chiropractors & Allied Professions Board
PO Box 17055
0027 Groenkloof
South Africa
Tel 1246 6455

UK and EIRE

British Complementary Medicine Association
St Charles Hospital
Exmoor Street
London W10 6DZ
Tel 0181 964 1205
Fax 0181 964 1207

British Diabetic Association
10 Queen Anne Street
London W1M OBD
Tel 0171 323 1531
Fax 0171 637 3644

British Holistic Medical Association
Trust House
Royal Shrewsbury Hospital (South)
Shrewsbury
Shropshire SY3 8XF
Tel 01743 261155
Fax 01743 3536373

Council for Complementary & Alternative Medicine
179 Gloucester Place
London NW1 6DX
Tel 0171 724 9103
Fax 0171 724 5330

Health Education Authority
Hamilton House
Mabledon Place
London WC1H 9TX
Tel 0171 383 3833
Fax 0171 387 0550

Institute for Complementary Medicine
PO Box 194
London SE16 1QZ
Tel 0171 237 5165
Fax 0171 237 5175

Irish Diabetic Association
76 Lower Gardiner Street
Dublin 1, Eire
Tel/fax 353 136 3022

Yoga Biomedical Trust
PO Box 140
Cambridge
CB1 1PU

APPENDIX B

Useful further reading

Aromatherapy: Massage with Essential Oils, Christine Wildwood (Element UK/USA, 1991)

Book of Stress Survival, Alixa Kirsta (Unwin, UK, 1986)

Complete Natural Health Consultant, Michael van Straten (Ebury Press, UK, 1986)

Counselling People with Diabetes, Richard Shillitoe (British Psychological Society, UK, 1994)

The Diabetes Handbook, John Day (British Diabetic Association, UK, 1986)

Encylopaedia of Natural Medicine, Michael Murray and Joseph Pizzorno (Optima, UK, 1994)

Essential Diabetic Cookbook, Azmina Govindji and Jill Myers (British Diabetic Association, 1994)

Family Guide to Homoeopathy, Andrew Lockie (Hamish Hamilton, UK, 1990)

Fitness Book for People with Diabetes, W Guyton Hornsby (American Diabetes Association, 1994)

Learning to Live Well with Diabetes, ed Cheryl Weller (DCI Publishing, USA, 1991)

Mothers, Babies and Disease in Later Life, D J P Barker (BMJ Publishing, UK, 1994)

Optimum Nutrition Workbook, Patrick Holford (ION Press, UK, 1988)

Parenting a Diabetic Child, Gloria Loring (Lowell House, USA, 1993)

Reader's Digest Family Guide to Alternative Medicine, ed Patrick Pietroni (Reader's Digest Association, UK/USA, 1991)

So Your Child Has Diabetes, Bonnie Estridge and Jo Davies (British Diabetic Association, 1993)

Treatment for Diabetic Neuropathy: A New Approach, ed David Horrobin (Churchill Livingstone, UK/USA, 1992)

Yoga for Common Ailments, R Nagarathna, H R Nagendra and Robin Monro (Gaia Books, UK, 1990)

Yoga Made Easy, Desmond Dunne (Souvenir Press, UK/Prentice-Hall, USA, 1994)

Index

THE NATURAL WAY SERIES

Increasing numbers of people worldwide are falling victim to illnesses which modern medicine, for all its technical advances, seems often powerless to prevent – and sometimes actually causes. To help with these so-called 'diseases of civilization' more and more people are turning to 'natural' medicine for an answer. The *Natural Way* series aims to offer clear, practical and reliable guidance to the safest, gentlest and most effective treatments available – and so to give sufferers and their families the information they need to make their own choices about the most suitable treatments.

Titles in the Natural Way *series*